UNFOLDING
HEALTH ASSESSMENT
CASE STUDIES
FOR THE STUDENT NURSE

SECOND EDITION

FACILITATOR GUIDE

KRISTI MAYNARD, EdD, APRN, FNP-BC, CNE

ANDREA ADIMANDO, DNP, MSN, MS, APRN, PMHNP-BC, BCIM

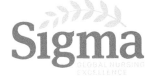

Sigma Theta Tau International Honor Society of Nursing (Sigma) is a nonprofit organization whose mission is developing nurse leaders anywhere to improve healthcare everywhere. Founded in 1922, Sigma has more than 135,000 active members in over 100 countries and territories. Members include practicing nurses, instructors, researchers, policymakers, entrepreneurs, and others. Sigma's more than 540 chapters are located at more than 700 institutions of higher education throughout Armenia, Australia, Botswana, Brazil, Canada, Chile, Colombia, Croatia, England, Eswatini, Finland, Ghana, Hong Kong, Ireland, Israel, Italy, Jamaica, Japan, Jordan, Kenya, Lebanon, Malawi, Mexico, the Netherlands, Nigeria, Pakistan, Philippines, Portugal, Puerto Rico, Scotland, Singapore, South Africa, South Korea, Sweden, Taiwan, Tanzania, Thailand, the United States, and Wales. Learn more at www.sigmanursing.org.

Sigma Theta Tau International
550 West North Street
Indianapolis, IN, USA 46202

To request a review copy for course adoption, order additional books, buy in bulk, or purchase for corporate use, contact Sigma Marketplace at 888.654.4968 (US/Canada toll-free), +1.317.687.2256 (International), or solutions@sigmamarketplace.org.

To request author information, or for speaker or other media requests, contact Sigma Marketing at 888.634.7575 (US/Canada toll-free) or +1.317.634.8171 (International).

ISBN:	9781646482801
EPUB ISBN:	9781646481798
PDF ISBN:	9781646481781

Publisher: Dustin Sullivan	**Managing Editor:** Carla Hall
Acquisitions Editor: Emily Hatch	**Publications Specialist:** Todd Lothery
Development Editor: Jillmarie Leeper Sycamore	**Project Editor:** Jillmarie Leeper Sycamore
Cover Designer: Rebecca Batchelor	**Copy Editor:** Todd Lothery
Interior Design/Page Layout: Bumpy Design	**Proofreader:** Todd Lothery

About the Authors

Kristi Maynard, EdD, APRN, FNP-BC, CNE, is an American Nurses Credentialing Center (ANCC) board-certified advanced practice registered nurse in the specialty area of family practice (FNP). She also achieved certification through the National League for Nursing as a certified nurse educator (CNE). She received her BSN from Mount Saint Mary College in Newburgh, New York, and her MSN from Fairfield University in Fairfield, Connecticut.

She began her career in nursing more than 15 years ago as a medical intensive care nurse. After graduating with her MSN, she entered full-time practice as an FNP in the primary care environment. She remains active in clinical practice in her independently owned and operated primary care practice. Currently, she is an Associate Professor of Nursing at Southern Connecticut State University and the lead family nurse practitioner faculty for their FNP program. She teaches in both the graduate and undergraduate nursing programs with a course load focused on health assessment, health assessment lab, pathophysiology, and pharmacology. In addition to her authorship, she contracts as an editorial consultant for nursing and nurse practitioner test bank content.

Andrea Adimando, DNP, MSN, MS, APRN, PMHNP-BC, BCIM, is an Associate Professor of Nursing and Director of the MSN program at Southern Connecticut State University. She is an ANCC board-certified psychiatric-mental health nurse practitioner (PMHNP-BC) and a former pediatric medical-surgical nurse. She earned a bachelor's degree in behavioral neuroscience from Lehigh University in 2003 and a master of science in nursing from Yale School of Nursing in 2006. She later earned a master of science in human nutrition from the University of Bridgeport in 2012 and a DNP from Chatham University in 2014.

In addition to her clinical practice, Adimando has published several peer-reviewed articles and presented at local and national conferences on her research interests. These include complementary and alternative therapies, multimodal educational strategies for nursing students, and compassion fatigue in nurses. She has also previously served as the Vice Chairperson on the ANCC's content expert panel for the PMHNP board certification exam, as well as a member of the panel for eight years. Recently, she received the ANCC's prestigious Certified Nurse Award for her contributions as a PMHNP in Connecticut.

Adimando has over 15 years of pediatric and psychiatric nursing experience and continues to practice as a PMHNP in various levels of care across Connecticut. Within her previous positions in emergency psychiatry, inpatient and outpatient psychiatry, her private practice, and pediatric medical-surgical settings, she focused on the integration and interdependence of physical and mental health. The health assessment skills she acquired through this expansive background allow her to apply real-life clinical scenarios and relevant expertise to her teaching of health assessment to BSN and MSN students.

Special Note to Readers

Here at Sigma, we realize that language is constantly evolving. The meaning of a word often changes over time, some words become obsolete, and some terms that were once acceptable may become controversial or even offensive, depending on the context or circumstances. We have made every effort to make language choices that are inclusive and not offensive. Should you identify words in this book that you believe negatively impact a group or groups of people, please reach out to us at Publications@SigmaNursing.org.

Table of Contents

Introduction

As nurse educators, we appreciate the effort it takes to keep students engaged in active learning. We hope this text will become an indispensable tool for your health assessment course planning. In this resource guide, we provide you with a snapshot of the contents of each chapter, along with recommendations for when each chapter might be most useful in your curriculum. To further enhance student learning and aid in the development of an immersive lesson plan, we provide discussion prompts and activities for each chapter to enrich the classroom experience. Thank you for choosing this facilitator guide for your students.

CHAPTER 1

Introduction to the Unfolding Case Study

This chapter reviews the value of integrating unfolding case studies as a routine method for studying nursing content. Often, a student will discredit or question the value of an activity if they cannot recognize the potential value. This chapter explains why unfolding case studies are a preferred study method to master complex concepts and foster skills of critical appraisal and dynamic response. If the student can understand the "why" and recognize the learning objectives, they are more likely to fully engage in the learning activity.

The advantages of working with unfolding case studies include:

- Provides more information about the patient and the patient's progress
- Begins with basic concepts and layers on more complex concepts as the case builds
- Encourages anticipating potential changes in patient status
- Develops clinical reasoning skills
- Utilizes low-fidelity simulation, which doesn't require a high-tech lab or mannequins
- Engages active learning

When to introduce this chapter: This chapter should be assigned prior to the assignment of the case studies in this text. This chapter is intended to be foundational and highlight the value and usefulness of the text.

Many of the chapters end with a worksheet (see Sample Worksheet at the end of this chapter). The worksheet contains prompts to direct learners' thoughts and help them identify areas of strength and weakness. Encourage students to use these worksheets to realistically evaluate their performance on the case. Self-evaluation is a valuable tool for personal growth.

Best Practices for Students Working With Unfolding Case Studies

Read each case carefully.

Put the book down for a few seconds after reading a new section of the vignette (the case) and think about how what you just read will affect your patient. How does this influence your plan of care? What are your priorities for care? Have your priorities changed based on the information you just read?

Don't jump ahead to the practice questions.

Be thoughtful about the patient scenario and consider the details you have been presented. Health assessment is about taking in the subjective and objective information that you gather and formulating priorities and a plan based on evidence-based best practice for patient care.

Read the questions carefully.

Underline key components of the question and then carefully read through the options. Think. It. Through. Simplify the question in your own words to make it more manageable (keeping scrap paper close by is helpful).

Read through the question rationale.

Take the time to read and understand why your selection was correct or incorrect. Make notes or comments on the page that help you identify and retain key pieces of information that may be helpful in your future studies. If you read a rationale and still find yourself uncertain about content or a concept, look it up! Use your textbook or an evidence-based search engine to get more information on what you are investigating.

Look through a new lens.

After you have completed the guidance questions, go back to the previous section of the vignette and read through it again. Now that you have acquired new knowledge, were there key elements in the patient description that might have led you to prioritize this patient differently?

Think ahead and take a moment to ask, "What if?"

Based on the current state and trajectory of your patient, what do you anticipate may happen to this patient in the future? How might that affect your nursing priorities or care?

Set yourself up for success!

Don't get discouraged or frustrated if you don't know the answer to a question. This is a tool for learning; it is not expected that you will answer every question perfectly. The questions are intended to provide practice with NCLEX-style questions while introducing relevant content.

Class Discussion Prompts

What is the value of active learning versus passive learning when considering a study plan?

Why is self-reflection so valuable?

What are some methods of self-reflection you use to enhance your learning?

Class Activity

Pair students and ask them to locate one evidence-based article (peer-reviewed journal) that explores the value of self-reflection in nursing. Pairs will summarize the article and present a brief summary to the class.

 Note

The following sample worksheet is included at the end of many chapters in the textbook but only reproduced once here in the facilitator guide.

Based on my initial assessment, I thought:

_____

_____

_____

Based on my revised/informed assessment, I now know:

_____

_____

_____

A nursing priority for this patient would be _____

because _____

After completing this chapter, something I have learned is:

_____

_____

_____

After completing this chapter, something I need more clarity on is:

_____

_____

_____

After completing this chapter, something else I want to learn is:

_____

_____

_____

CHAPTER 2

Introduction to the Nursing Process

This chapter reviews the steps of the nursing process. It offers guidance on rationale application of the steps of the nursing process and describes how useful the nursing process is in both completing the case studies in this text and evaluating NCLEX-style questions, including NextGen formatted questions. In addition, this chapter reviews NANDA criteria for the formulation of a nursing diagnosis.

The nursing process (see Figure 2.1) consists of five basic steps (Potter et al., 2017):

1. Assessment
2. Diagnosis
3. Planning (sometimes referred to as Outcomes and Planning)
4. Implementation
5. Evaluation

Understanding the nursing process is key to critical thinking and problem-solving in nursing practice. Each of these steps is described in detail in this chapter and also referenced in Chapter 3 in regard to preparing to answer NCLEX-style questions. However, for the purposes of this book, the primary focus is on the assessment phase of the nursing process.

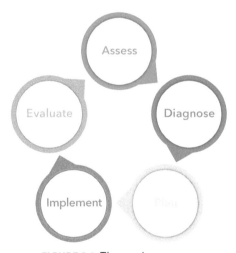

FIGURE 2.1 The nursing process.

When identifying and validating a nursing diagnosis, it is important to ensure that (NANDA International, 2018):

- The majority of the defining characteristics and/or risk factors are present in the patient.
- The etiological factors for the diagnosis are evident in the patient.
- You have validated the diagnosis with the patient/family or with a nurse peer (when possible).

Table 2.1 shows a series of nursing diagnoses for which the nurse has planned goals and expected outcomes for a patient who is postoperative.

TABLE 2.1 Nursing Diagnoses, Goals, and Expected Outcomes for the Postoperative Patient

Nursing Diagnoses	Goals	Outcomes Expected
Pain related to surgery	Mrs. Radiant will achieve pain relief by day of discharge.	Pt reports pain at a level of < 4 by day of discharge.
		Pt transfers from bed to chair with no increase in pain in 48 hours.
Knowledge deficit related to impending discharge	Mrs. Radiant will express understanding of postoperative risks. Mrs. Radiant will verbalize self-care needs.	Pt verbalizes home activity restrictions by day of discharge.
		Pt verbalizes knowledge and demonstrates skill of cleaning incision by day of discharge.
		Pt describes risks for infection within one day of surgery.
Risk for infection	Mrs. Radiant will remain infection-free while in the hospital.	Patient remains afebrile while in the hospital.
		Patient's incision shows no signs of infection.
		Pt incisional area shows signs of healing and closure by day of discharge.

(Adapted from Potter et al., 2017)

As shown in Table 2.1, all goals are directly related to the nursing diagnoses and are measurable and attainable. If goals are not attainable, the care plan will not be successful, and the objectives will not be met. This often requires critical thinking and careful reassessment to achieve. The expected outcomes also match the diagnoses and the goals, and they should be reasonable and measurable as well.

When to introduce this chapter: Just as with Chapter 1, this chapter is intended to offer foundational information that will guide the student's thought process as they work through the case studies. It should be introduced prior to beginning the cases.

Class Discussion Prompts

Do you view the nursing process as linear or cyclic? Why?

In your current experience as a student nurse, name a scenario or situation you have observed and describe how the nursing process was applied to improve the patient outcome.

Class Activity

Provide the students with a brief patient scenario. Ask them to write a NANDA-style nursing diagnosis based on the information provided.

REFERENCES

NANDA International. (2018). *Nursing diagnoses: Definitions and classification*. https://nanda.org/publications-resources/publications/nanda-international-nursing-diagnoses/

Potter, P. A., Perry, A. G., & Stockert, P. (2017). *Fundamentals of nursing* (9th ed.). Elsevier, Inc.

CHAPTER 3

Answering NCLEX-Style Questions

This chapter reviews the current standards of the NCLEX exam. The current NCLEX test plan and content distribution are discussed and presented with visual aids for quick reference. The chapter provides an in-depth approach to the interpretation of the various styles of NCLEX questions and discusses tips for rationale answer selection, including nursing concepts such as Maslow's hierarchy of needs and the prioritization of the ABCs (airway, breathing, circulation).

The Anatomy of NCLEX Questions

Prior to NextGen, there were five styles of NCLEX questions:

1. Multiple choice
2. Multiple response
3. Hotspot
4. Fill-in-the-blank
5. Drag-and-drop/ordered response

The chapter provides examples of each of these types of questions, including a rationale for the correct answer.

New Styles of Questions in the NextGen NCLEX

The NextGen exam has added the following four types of questions:

1. Case studies
2. Stand-alone
3. Bowtie
4. Extended multiple response

The chapter provides examples of each of these types of questions, including a rationale for the correct answer.

What Makes an NCLEX-Style Question Unique?

NCLEX-style questions are generally worded in a way that requires analysis and interpretation before even attempting to answer. Questions are known for providing more information than necessary, requiring the test taker to discern what is relevant and what is not. A question stem may prompt students to select an option that is *not* correct or *most* correct, and if they miss those key differentiating terms while taking the exam, they will likely select the wrong answer.

It is also a possibility for a multiple-choice question to have more than one correct answer. The challenge is to choose which item is most correct based on the stem of the question. These nuances may prove challenging for a test taker who is unfamiliar with the NCLEX format.

NCLEX Test Plan

The test plan is revised and republished every three years, ensuring that content is aligned with current practice and existing nurse practice acts. The newest test plan is effective as of April 2023 (NCSBN, 2022) and therefore will be the test plan that is discussed within this chapter.

The NCLEX test plan structure is devised to be in line with the contents of the NCLEX examination, to provide a guide for educators and students when preparing for this examination. Figure 3.1 illustrates the NCLEX-RN test plan.

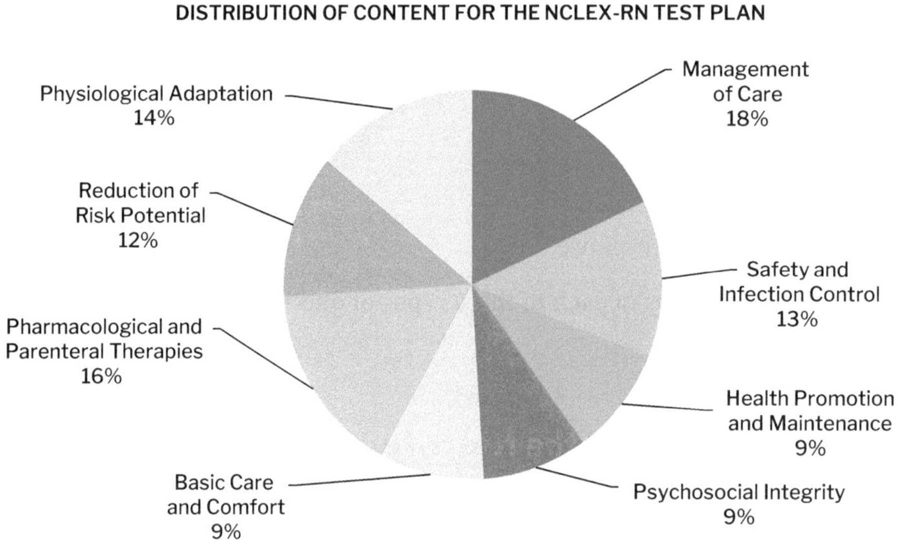

DISTRIBUTION OF CONTENT FOR THE NCLEX-RN TEST PLAN

- Physiological Adaptation 14%
- Reduction of Risk Potential 12%
- Pharmacological and Parenteral Therapies 16%
- Basic Care and Comfort 9%
- Management of Care 18%
- Safety and Infection Control 13%
- Health Promotion and Maintenance 9%
- Psychosocial Integrity 9%

FIGURE 3.1 NCLEX-RN test plan (NCSBN, 2022).

The Client Needs Framework

The NextGen NCLEX is structured using the "client needs" framework "because it provides a universal structure for defining nursing actions and competencies and focuses on clients in all settings" (NCSBN, 2022, p. 7). *Client needs* is a concept that is divided into four major categories and further into subcategories. These are (NCSBN, 2022, p. 9):

- Safe and effective care environment
  - Management of care
  - Safety and infection control
- Health promotion and maintenance
- Psychosocial integrity

- Physiological integrity
  - Basic care and comfort
  - Pharmacological and parenteral therapies
  - Reduction of risk potential
  - Physiological adaption

Additional NCLEX Categories

In addition to the major categories of client needs, the NCLEX-RN also integrates concepts from nursing prerequisite coursework, including:

- Social sciences such as psychology
- Biological sciences such as anatomy & physiology and microbiology
- Physical sciences such as physics and chemistry

Additional important nursing concepts that are interwoven within the client need categories and will be important for students to have mastered prior to entering the examination include:

- The nursing process
- Caring
- Communication and documentation
- Teaching and learning
- Culture and spirituality
- Clinical judgment

Clinical judgment is a new addition to the NextGen NCLEX and may be posed as a case study or as an individual item. Case studies, also new to NextGen, contain six items that correlate with one client presentation, share client information in an unfolding manner, and address the following components of clinical judgment (NCSBN, 2022, p. 8):

Recognize cues: Identify relevant and important information from different sources (e.g., medical history, vital signs).

Analyze cues: Organize and connect the recognized cues to the client's clinical presentation.

Prioritize hypotheses: Evaluate and prioritize hypotheses (urgency, likelihood, risk, difficulty, time constraints, etc.).

Generate solutions: Identify expected outcomes and use hypotheses to define a set of interventions for the expected outcomes.

Take action: Implement the solutions that address the highest priority.

Evaluate outcomes: Compare observed outcomes to expected outcomes.

Techniques for Mastering NCLEX-Style Questions

NCLEX-style questions are highly complex and often involve a new way of thinking and synthesizing multiple levels of information.

One of the major differences between the NCLEX-RN and other certification exams is that there may be more than one correct answer to the question. Often, the test taker is tasked with selecting the "best" answer (or answers, if a select-all-that-apply question) from a series of options. Here are a series of techniques students can utilize when answering any type of NCLEX question, including those that require them to choose the best out of a series of options.

Read the Question Carefully and Thoughtfully

Although this may sound silly and obvious, many students do not fully read the stem of the question. The *stem* is the text body of the question that lets readers know what is being asked of them and presents all the information they need to answer the question.

Before jumping to the answer choices, which may result in an impulsive or ill-informed selection, it is important the test takers ask themselves before and after reading the question stem (and before looking at the answer choices!):

- What is this question really asking of me?

  Is it asking you to simply recall and regurgitate knowledge, apply a concept, or prioritize nursing interventions? Is it asking you to act according to the nursing process?

- What information do I need to answer this question?

  This may include information in the question stem (e.g., a lab value, an assessment finding, a patient complaint, etc.) or information that you have learned throughout your nursing program (e.g., normal range of lab values, the nursing process, etc.).

- Have I read into this question and added factors that are not important or not valid?

  Often, exam takers will make a question harder than it actually is by assuming information that was not in fact given or making a patient sicker than they really are by overthinking the question. Be sure you are not doing this before you move on to looking at the answer choices, as this will help you be less likely to choose the distractors that may be geared toward "overthinkers."

Consider Your "ABCs"

The "ABCs," as frequently referred to in nursing school, are **A**irway, **B**reathing, and **C**irculation. The authors of this book encourage considering the "S" for **S**afety, after they have considered A, B, and C. Considering the ABCs may help test takers in priority-style questions that ask students to determine which would be the "next" or "immediate" or "priority" action—all common terms seen in question stems that are trying to glean this information. Each term is outlined in Table 3.1.

TABLE 3.1 The ABCs

Airway	Ensure the patient has a clear or "patent" (usable, functioning) airway.
Breathing	You need to be sure the patient is breathing adequately.
Circulation	You need to be sure your patient's blood is properly flowing, circulating, and perfusing their body.
Safety	Once you have established that the patient has a patent airway, is breathing adequately, and circulating, you should always consider their safety before moving on to other priorities or interventions.

Without these functions being intact, the patient cannot function or survive, so these are your priority assessments for all patients, *in this order.*

Remember the Nursing Process

As covered in Chapter 2, the nursing process is pivotal to nursing education and nursing practice. One of the strategies for answering NCLEX questions involves applying and differentiating aspects of the nursing process.

As mentioned earlier in this chapter, many NCLEX questions require the nurse to prioritize patient care based on information given and prior knowledge obtained in nursing school. If a question does not directly relate to the ABCs, the nursing process may be the next best framework from which to formulate an answer.

To help evaluate which stage of the nursing process a question is geared toward, the following are some general characteristics that questions may have, depending on which phase of the process they are alluding to:

1. **Assessment:** These typically will be questions that involve collecting, confirming, and communicating data about a patient's condition. Look for keywords that may be referring to an assessment technique or need. However, if it is an emergent situation, be sure to note whether an intervention might be warranted (remember your ABCs) prior to initiating or completing an assessment.

2. **Diagnosis:** This phase, also called *analysis,* involves interpreting data (collected during the assessment phase) and making clinical judgments based on this interpretation. These can be very challenging questions as a result of the higher-level thinking required to answer them.

3. **Outcomes and planning:** This phase involves determining the expected clinical outcomes for your patient and planning how you will care for this patient to achieve said outcomes. If you do not yet have your assessment data or your diagnostic clinical judgment, it is nearly impossible to approach this step. Questions that involve creating a plan of care, determining outcome goals, and prioritizing problems when planning care are likely referring to this phase of the process.

4. **Implementation:** These questions almost always involve a nursing action, typically geared toward meeting the goals of the patient care plan. Remember that these questions are looking for a nursing intervention or other implementation strategy and not a medical one (though medical ones make great distractors). Anything involving communicating and/or documenting these interventions would also fall under this question category.

5. **Evaluation:** Questions about this phase of the nursing process usually involve comparing actual outcomes for a patient to the anticipated outcomes and determining whether the patient has responded appropriately to the care in place. Sometimes the evaluation will lead to a change in implementation, so these types of questions may be closely linked.

The most important thing to remember is that the nursing process is an "order of operations," so to speak. That is, you must assess before you diagnose, plan before you implement, etc. So, if you see a prioritization or a "next step" type of question, ask yourself, "What phase of the nursing process is this testing?" If you have not fully assessed yet, you should not be choosing an answer that involves diagnosing or intervening, for example.

Remember Maslow's Hierarchy of Needs

Another important conceptual framework that will undoubtedly show up on the NCLEX-RN is Maslow's hierarchy of needs theory. Essentially, it is a way to categorize patient needs in a prioritized fashion. The hierarchy within this theory is displayed in Figure 3.2.

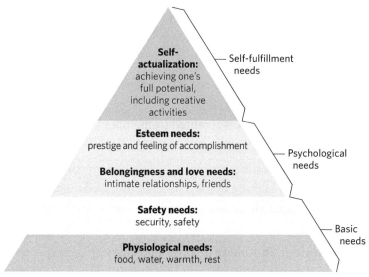

FIGURE 3.2 Maslow's hierarchy of needs.

With this theory, a person's physiological needs take precedence over all others. If their physiological needs are not met—basic things such as food, shelter, sleep—then the other needs cannot be adequately addressed. Therefore, when answering a question that may involve any level of patient need, Maslow's hierarchy should always be considered. If an answer choice addresses physiological needs, it is most likely the correct answer.

When to introduce this chapter: Ideally this chapter is assigned prior to beginning the case studies. It may also be useful as a test prep guide/reference for students struggling to answer NCLEX-style questions.

Class Discussion Prompts

After reviewing the different types of NCLEX questions, what do you think is the most challenging and why?

How might you adapt your study habits to better prepare for this style of question?

Class Activity

Preparation: Select or write five sample NCLEX-style questions.

Activity: Ask students to work in pairs to review the questions and highlight pertinent information in the body of the question. Have students summarize the question in their own words, using "What is the question asking of me?" as a prompt. Students will then select the answer and provide a brief rationale to explain why each answer is correct or incorrect.

Share results with the class and discuss.

REFERENCE

National Council of State Boards of Nursing. (2022). *Next Generation NCLEX-RN® test plan.* https://www.ncsbn.org/public-files/2023_RN_Test%20Plan_English_FINAL.pdf

CHAPTER 4

Introduction to Approaching the Patient Interview

This chapter reviews the approach to the patient interview, including common pitfalls, and focuses on the importance of building nurse-patient relationships. It explores the function of common interview methods such as open and closed questions, when focused versus comprehensive assessments are appropriate, and commonly used mnemonics to guide the interview such as PQRSTU.

Getting Started

For most patient encounters, the interview will take place during the first meeting with the patient. This can be when a patient is being evaluated in the emergency department for an acute complaint or when they are presenting for their routine healthcare at an outpatient environment. The order and urgency of the interview may vary depending on the acuity of the patient and the care setting, but the steps are the same.

When preparing to interview a patient, students should understand that they are establishing a new relationship. How they approach their interactions with this individual will impact how receptive they are to answering the questions, especially personal ones. Establishing a relationship of transparency and respect is a critical step in the interview process:

- As best you can, make the interview environment private and comfortable.
- Position yourself in a manner that promotes conversation and reduces the feeling of inequitable power distribution:
  - At eye level with patient
  - Unobstructed view
  - Speaking directly with eye contact
- Be professionally dressed and groomed.
- Deliver culturally competent care:
  - Ask for the patient's primary language and have a certified medical interpreter available if needed.
  - Be aware that the patient's culture and/or religion may affect their health beliefs.
  - Accommodate any cultural preferences as to the patient's gender, age, or religion.
- Introduce yourself and your role in their care.

- Ask the patient how they would like to be addressed (first or last name; pronouns).
- Explain why any sensitive questions are necessary.
- Reassure and support the patient if they feel awkward answering sensitive questions.

Asking Questions

There are two main question formats: open- and closed-ended questions. An *open-ended question* is formatted to allow the patient to provide a more detailed narrative response, while a *closed-ended question* usually requires a simple answer, like "yes" or "no." There are times when one style of question might be more appropriate to use. In an emergency when you need to gather specific information quickly, the closed-ended approach is usually a better choice since you can ask direct questions quickly. On the other hand, the open-ended approach is more helpful when you are collecting a comprehensive patient health history.

Focused Versus Comprehensive Interviewing

Depending on why the patient is seeking care, a focused or comprehensive approach to interviewing might be more appropriate. A focused interview focuses only on the details of the patient's presenting complaint and does not ask for information that is not relevant to why they are seeking care. As an example, if a patient was consulting with their primary care clinic because they suspected they had an ear infection, the nurse would not ask about a family history of cardiac disease. On the other hand, if a new patient is presenting to their primary care provider for an annual physical exam, the nurse would collect a comprehensive history because they need an inclusive picture of the patient's health. Time may also be a factor when choosing your approach. In an urgent situation, a brief, focused exam might be more suitable than an extended, comprehensive interview.

Using PQRSTU to Aid in Data Collection

When collecting information about symptoms or a complaint, the PQRSTU mnemonic is a helpful tool to organize your questions. PQRSTU stands for:

P—Provoking/Palliative

This includes asking what makes the symptom better or worse.

Q—Quality

This looks to gather a description of the symptom.

R—Region/Radiation

This identifies the location of the symptom and whether other symptoms are associated with it.

S—Severity

This speaks to how severe the symptom is or how badly it is impacting the patient. We often see a 0–10 numeric scale used for this aspect.

T—Timing

This would include when the symptom started, how long it has been present, and also if it has ever been experienced before.

U—Understanding

This looks to capture the patient's perception of what is happening and can provide valuable insight into what the patient is experiencing.

Common Pitfalls

Even the most seasoned nurse can fall victim to some of the common interviewing pitfalls. Being mindful and present during the interview process can help you avoid some of these practices that can otherwise impact the effectiveness of the patient interview:

- Be mindful of your body language.
- Avoid leading or judgmental wording.
- Be careful to avoid the use of jargon or technical language.
- When working with patients who are disabled, elderly, or adolescent, direct questions to the patient directly, not to their caregiver whenever possible.
- If you must communicate with the caregiver, make sure the caregiver is HIPAA-compliant and note in the chart that the primary source of data was not the patient but a caregiver.
- Provide culturally competent care.

When to introduce this chapter: This chapter is intended to offer foundational information that will guide students' thought process as they work through the case studies. It should be introduced prior to beginning the cases.

Class Discussion Prompts

First, review the differences between open- and closed-ended questions.

As a group, present students with a brief description of a presenting complaint—for example, a headache or chest pain. Ask students to work in pairs to determine one open-ended and one closed-ended question to gather information for each element of the PQRSTU mnemonic.

After each group is finished, return to the larger group to discuss the challenges of formatting questions both ways. For each element of the mnemonic, what do they think they would prefer to use for the scenario—the open or closed variation of the interview question? Why?

An example might be:

For P for provokes, an open-ended question might be: "Tell me what makes the pain worse." A closed-ended question might be: "Does anything make the pain worse?"

Class Activity

Prepare slips of paper with a variety of different presenting complaints—for example, a headache or chest pain. Place the slips of paper into a bowl and break students into pairs. Circulate the room and have each student take a slip from the bowl—this will be their presenting complaint in the role-playing activity. If you would like, you can give the students a few moments to use their text and sources to determine how they will choose to portray the complaint.

After students are prepared, they will take turns interviewing one another with the goal of completing a focused interview in 10 minutes. Students will decide who will be the patient first and who will be the nurse. Set a timer for 10 minutes. When time has elapsed, the students will switch roles. When the activity is over, return to the larger group to discuss what was challenging about this exercise. What question styles did they find themselves using? How might they change their approach in the future?

CHAPTER 5

Vital Sign Assessment

This chapter reviews basic techniques for obtaining a full set of vital signs with nursing considerations for the pediatric and adult populations and provides opportunities to apply this knowledge.

Vital signs are an integral part of performing a nursing assessment. Vital signs can be performed quickly and yield valuable information about the hemodynamic status of the patient. A full set of vital signs includes blood pressure, pulse, respiratory rate, temperature, and oxygen saturation.

Blood Pressure

Routine measurement of blood pressure is important for identifying trends and assessing for hypertension or hypotension (Muntner et al., 2019). Nurses routinely assess blood pressure as an indicator of hemodynamic stability to evaluate the effectiveness of medications and various interventions. The equipment needed to obtain a noninvasive blood pressure reading is a sphygmomanometer and stethoscope.

Proper Technique

There are several important nursing considerations when obtaining a blood pressure reading to ensure accuracy in the measurement:

- Cuff size
- Cuff placement
- Patient position
- Patient considerations

Procedure

Before beginning with obtaining a blood pressure measurement, explain the procedure to the patient. Once you have determined the correct cuff size and the patient is positioned optimally, you can proceed with obtaining the blood pressure measurement:

1. To determine the patient's estimated blood pressure, place the blood pressure cuff on the patient's arm and palpate the brachial artery. Inflate the blood pressure cuff while simultaneously palpating the brachial artery, and take note on the manometer when the pulse becomes no longer palpable. When obtaining the blood pressure, the blood pressure cuff should be inflated 30 mmHG higher than the measurement noted when the pulse was no longer palpable (Muntner et al., 2019). For example, if the brachial pulse was no longer palpable at 120 mmHG, the blood pressure cuff should be inflated to 150 mmHG when obtaining the blood pressure measurement.

2. To obtain an auscultatory blood pressure reading, put the cuff in place on the patient's upper arm and palpate the location of the brachial artery, then place the diaphragm of the stethoscope over the brachial artery.

3. Secure the dial on the manometer so that the cuff may be inflated, and then proceed with inflating the cuff to the estimated systolic measurement. Once the cuff is inflated, proceed with opening the dial on the air release valve slowly. The manometer should decrease by 2–3 mmHg per second to allow for accuracy in auscultation (Muntner et al., 2019).

4. The sounds that are heard when auscultating the blood pressure are referred to as *Korotkoff sounds.* The first audible sound is the systolic pressure. Continue to deflate the cuff by slowly releasing the air release valve and take note of the last sound heard—this is the diastolic pressure. The systolic and diastolic pressures are recorded in mmHg—for example, 110/70 mmHG.

See Tables 5.1 and 5.2 for normal and abnormal blood pressure measurements for adult and pediatric populations.

TABLE 5.1 Adult Blood Pressure Measurements

	Systolic Pressure	Diastolic Pressure
Hypotension	< 90	
Normal	< 120	< 80
Elevated blood pressure	120–129	< 80
Hypertension (Stage 1)	130–139	80–89
Hypertension (Stage 2)	> 140	> 90

(Whelton et al., 2018)

It is important to note that systolic pressures > 180 and diastolic pressures > 120 in the absence of symptoms such as chest or back discomfort or neurological changes are referred to as *hypertensive urgency* (American Heart Association, 2023b). Systolic pressures > 180 and diastolic pressures > 120 with symptoms of chest or back discomfort or neurological changes are referred to as *hypertensive crisis* and require immediate intervention (American Heart Association, 2023b).

TABLE 5.2 Pediatric Blood Pressure Measurements

	Systolic Pressure	Diastolic Pressure
Neonate	67–84	35–53
Infant	72–104	37–56
Toddler	86–106	42–83
Preschool age (3–5)	89–112	46–72
School age (6–9)	97–115	57–76
Preadolescent (10–12)	102–120	61–80
Adolescent (12–15)	110–131	64–83

(American Heart Association, 2020)

Among pediatric populations, the diagnosis of normal blood pressure is defined as systolic and diastolic pressures < 90th percentile when considering age, sex, and height percentiles (Flynn et al., 2017). High blood pressure is defined as systolic and diastolic pressures >/= 95th percentile when taking into account age, sex, and height percentiles (Flynn et al., 2017).

Pulse

Pulse, also referred to as *heart rate*, is the measurement of how many times the heart beats every minute. Alterations in pulse can occur with a multitude of conditions. Establishing a baseline pulse rate allows the nurse to identify fluctuations in rate and rhythm and correlate the findings clinically.

The equipment needed to obtain a radial pulse is a watch with a second hand. The equipment needed to obtain an apical pulse is a stethoscope and a watch with a second hand.

Procedure

Before beginning with obtaining a pulse measurement, explain the procedure to the patient.

Pulses can be obtained in multiple places on the body; however, the most common places for obtaining a pulse measurement for vital signs is the radial artery or the apical pulse (Potter et al., 2022).

Radial pulse: To obtain a radial pulse assessment, place your first two fingertips on the radial artery, located thumb side on the lateral aspect of the wrist. A grooved area between the radial bone and the tendon in the wrist is the most optimal location for obtaining the pulse (Potter et al., 2022). Palpate for the radial artery until consistent pulsation is felt, and begin counting the pulsations for one full minute. The pulse is recorded in beats per minute (for example, 70 beats per minute).

Apical pulse: To obtain an apical pulse, place the diaphragm of the stethoscope on the patient's chest along the fifth intercostal space at the left midclavicular line (Potter et al., 2022). This location is referred to as the *point of maximal impulse* (PMI) and is clinically significant because this is the point correlating to the location of the apex of the heart, where cardiac sounds are heard most prominently (Potter et al., 2022).

When the PMI landmark has been located, auscultate heart sounds, and when consistent S1 and S2 ("lub dub") sounds are heard, begin counting the heart rate for one full minute (see Figure 5.1).

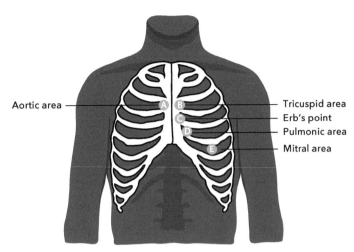

FIGURE 5.1 Cardiac auscultatory locations.

The apical pulse is recorded in beats per minute. Documentation should note that the pulse measurement was obtained apically. See Tables 5.3 and 5.4 for normal and abnormal pulse rates for adult and pediatric populations.

TABLE 5.3 **Adult Pulse Rates**

Normal	60-100 beats per minute
Bradycardic	< 60 beats per minute
Tachycardic	> 100 beats per minute

(American Heart Association, 2023a)

TABLE 5.4 **Pediatric Pulse Rates**

Neonatal	100-205
Infant	100-180
Toddler	98-140
Preschool	80-120
School age	75-118
Adolescent	60-100

(American Heart Association, 2020)

Respiratory Rate

Accuracy in measuring respiratory rate is critical because literature supports that alterations in respiratory rate are among the first signs that a patient's condition is deteriorating (Loughlin et al., 2018). Alterations in respiratory rate can occur in the setting of overwhelming infection, neurological disorders, anemia, metabolic syndromes, and as side effects to certain medications (Hill & Annesley, 2020). The equipment needed to obtain a respiratory rate is a watch with a second hand.

Procedure

It is advisable to avoid acknowledging to the patient that you are counting their respirations because the patient may alter their respiratory pattern (Potter et al., 2022). To obtain a respiratory rate measurement, your patient should be lying or sitting comfortably so that visualization of chest rise and fall can occur unobstructed. To measure respiratory rate, each chest rise and fall is counted as one respiration. Respirations should be counted for one full minute. Avoid shortcut methods such as counting respirations for 30 seconds and multiplying the number of respirations by 2, as this can lead to inaccuracy in measurement, especially in patients with abnormal patterns of breathing (i.e., Cheyne-Stokes respirations). See Tables 5.5 and 5.6 for normal and abnormal respiratory rates for adult and pediatric populations.

TABLE 5.5 Adult Respiratory Rates

Normal	12–20 breaths per minute
Bradypnea	< 12 breaths per minute
Tachypnea	> 20 breaths per minute

(Hill & Annesley, 2020)

TABLE 5.6 Pediatric Respiratory Rates

Infant	30–53 breaths per minute
Toddler	22–37 breaths per minute
Preschool	20–28 breaths per minute
School age	18–25 breaths per minute
Adolescent	12–20 breaths per minute

(American Heart Association, 2020)

Temperature

Body temperature can be influenced by several factors, including age, environmental exposures, hormonal fluctuations, exercise, stress, and site of temperature measurement (Geneva et al., 2019; Potter et al., 2022). Routine temperature measurement (see Table 5.7) can be valuable in the clinical setting for identifying a fever, which can indicate the potential presence of an infection.

Procedure

This chapter details the variations in the technique for obtaining a temperature measurement depending on the site chosen to obtain temperature and nursing considerations associated with each site, including illustrations showing proper placement of the temperature device. Procedures and illustrations shown are:

- Oral
- Axillary

- ◦ Temporal
- ◦ Tympanic
- ◦ Rectal

TABLE 5.7 Adult and Pediatric Temperature Measurement

Normal (average)	98.6° F/37° C
Fever	>/ 100.4° F/38° C
Hypothermia	</ 95° F/35° C

(American Academy of Pediatrics, 2020; Centers for Disease Control and Prevention, 2017)

Although the average normal temperature is 98.6°, a range of 97.7°–99.5° F is generally acceptable (Sapra et. al., 2023).

Pulse Oximetry

Measurement of pulse oximetry requires the use of a device called an *oximeter*, which yields two light-emitting diodes (LEDs), red and infrared light. When the device is clipped to the body, generally a fingertip, the lights pass through the body, and the absorption of these lights varies among blood that is oxygen-rich and blood that is oxygen-deficient. Oxygen-rich blood absorbs more infrared light, whereas oxygen-deficient blood allows more infrared light to pass through. The ratio of these two lights' absorption yields an estimation of the oxygen saturation of the blood, which is expressed as a percentage (Pesola & Sankari, 2023).

Procedure

To obtain an oxygen saturation measurement, place the oximeter on the part of the body that the device is indicated for use. Most pulse oximeters are designed to be placed on the fingertip. However, there are devices made specifically for earlobes, or adhesive bandage-style oximeters that can be taped to the finger or foot and are commonly used among pediatric populations. Ensure that placement of the oximeter is per manufacturer guidelines, as utilizing a device on an area of the body for which it is not intended can yield false measurements (Hlavin & Varty, 2022). Once the device is placed correctly, the device should be powered on, and the sensor should remain in place until a consistent waveform is established. Simultaneous assessment of the patient's radial pulse in comparison to the pulse measurement on the device can assist with checking accuracy. The measurement should be recorded as a percentage—for example, oxygen saturation of 98%.

Patient Considerations

There are several factors that can influence the accuracy of measuring an oxygen saturation, such as:

- ◦ The presence of nail polish on fingernails
- ◦ Alterations in skin temperature

- Low perfusion states
- Patient movement (Food and Drug Administration, 2021)
- Racial bias—specifically, that devices yield overestimations of oxygen saturation and pose a patient safety risk in the identification of low oxygen states (Rathod et al., 2022)

Normal oxygen saturation for both adults and children is 95%–100% (Cleveland Clinic, 2022; Mau et al., 2005).

In assessing oxygen saturation values, take into account the patient's underlying conditions and baseline oxygen saturation levels. Patients with chronic respiratory conditions may have patient-specific acceptable oxygen levels that are lower than normal. Knowledge of these patient-specific criteria is critical when assessing oxygen saturation levels to determine if the level is acceptable.

When to introduce this chapter: Introducing vital signs at the beginning of the health assessment course facilitates student understanding of what the normal ranges for vital signs are, how to obtain them, and concepts of early clinical judgment for how students might interpret or react to abnormal findings. Exposing students to this content early on allows for scaffolding of more complex topics as the course progresses.

Class Discussion Prompts

As a group, discuss possible causes of vital sign variation. For example:

What might cause a patient's blood pressure to become elevated?

How can we relate what we know about pathophysiology to why we see this change occur?

What might be some assessment finding we observe, subjectively and objectively, as a result of this change?

If we were to observe this finding, what terminology might we use to appropriately document our findings?

Introduce these prompts as part of a group discussion. Discuss each of the vital signs to explore the potential implications.

Class Activity

Obtaining a set of vital signs is a skill that can take time to master. In health assessment, we are not only focused on the ability to interpret but also the ability to execute the tactile skill. For this chapter, place students in groups of two or three and have them practice collecting a set of vital signs on their peers. Ideally, a dual-headed stethoscope is available so students working in triads can verify the accuracy of their peers' blood pressure readings. This method utilizes the element of reciprocal peer teaching, where students engage in active learning within their groups, even if you as the instructor are not immediately present as they practice the skill.

REFERENCES

American Academy of Pediatrics. (2020). *How to take your child's temperature.* https://www.healthychildren.org/English/health-issues/conditions/fever/Pages/How-to-Take-a-Childs-Temperature.aspx

American Heart Association (2020). *PALS digital reference cards.* https://shopcpr.heart.org/pals-digital-reference-card

American Heart Association. (2023a). *All about heart rate (pulse).* https://www.heart.org/en/health-topics/high-blood-pressure/the-facts-about-high-blood-pressure/all-about-heart-rate-pulse

American Heart Association. (2023b). *Hypertensive crisis: When you should call 911 for high blood pressure.* https://www.heart.org/en/health-topics/high-blood-pressure/understanding-blood-pressure-readings/hypertensive-crisis-when-you-should-call-911-for-high-blood-pressure

Centers for Disease Control and Prevention. (2017). *Definitions of symptoms for reportable illnesses.* https://www.cdc.gov/quarantine/air/reporting-deaths-illness/definitions-symptoms-reportable-illnesses.html#:~:text=CDC%20considers%20a%20person%20to,a%20history%20of%20feeling%20feverish

Cleveland Clinic (2022). *Blood oxygen level.* https://my.clevelandclinic.org/health/diagnostics/22447-blood-oxygen-level

Flynn, J., Kaelber, D., Smith, C., Blowey, D., Carroll, A., Daniels, S., de Ferranti, S., Dionne, J., Falkner, B., Flinn, S., Gidding, S., Goodwin, C., Leu, M., Powers, M., Rea, C., Samuels, J., Simasek, M., Thaker, V., & Urbina, E. (2017). Clinical practice guideline for screening and management of high blood pressure in children and adolescents. *Pediatrics, 140*(3), 1–72. https://doi.org/10.1542/peds.2017-1904

Food and Drug Administration. (2021). *Pulse oximeter accuracy and limitations: FDA safety communication.* https://www.fda.gov/medical-devices/safety-communications/pulse-oximeter-accuracy-and-limitations-fda-safety-communication#:~:text=Follow%20your%20health%20care%20provider%27s,and%20use%20of%20fingernail%20polish

Geneva, I., Cuzzo, B., Fazili, T. & Javaid, W. (2019). Normal body temperature: A systematic review. *Open Forum Infectious Diseases, 6*(4), 1–7. https://doi.org/10.1093/ofid/ofz032

Hill, B., & Annesley, S. (2020). Monitoring respiratory rate in adults. *British Journal of Nursing, 29*(1), 12–16. https://doi.org/10.12968/bjon.2020.29.1.12

Hlavin, D., & Varty, M. (2022). Improving patient safety by increasing staff knowledge of evidence-based pulse oximetry practices. *American Association of Critical Care Nurses, 42*(6), 1–6. https://aacnjournals.org/ccnonline/article/42/6/e1/31885/Improving-Patient-Safety-by-Increasing-Staff

Loughlin, P. C., Sebat, F., & Kellett, J. G. (2018). Respiratory rate: The forgotten vital sign—make it count! *The Joint Commission Journal on Quality and Patient Safety, 44*, 494–499. https://doi.org/10.1016/j.jcjq.2018.04.014

Mau, M., Yamasato, K., & Yamamoto, L. (2005). Normal oxygen saturation values in pediatric patients. *Hawaii Medical Journal, 64*, 42–45. https://www.researchgate.net/profile/Loren-Yamamoto/publication/7866114_Normal_oxygen_saturation_values_in_pediatric_patients/links/56b2b60508ae5ec4ed4b59de/Normal-oxygen-saturation-values-in-pediatric-patients?_tp=eyJjb250ZXh0Ijp7ImZpcnN0UGFnZSI6InBlYmxpY2F0aW9uIiwicGFnZSI6InBlYmxpY2F0aW9uIn19

Muntner, P., Shimbo, D., Carey, R., Charleston, J., Gaillard, T., Misra, S., Myers, M., Ogedegbe, G., Schwartz, J., Townsend, R., Urbina, E., Viera, A., White, W., & Jackson, W. (2019). Measurement of blood pressure in humans: A scientific statement from the American Heart Association. *Hypertension, 73*(5), 35–66. https://www.ahajournals.org/doi/10.1161/HYP.0000000000000087

Pesola, G. R., & Sankari, A. (2023). Oxygenation status and pulse oximeter analysis. *StatPearls.* https://www.ncbi.nlm.nih.gov/books/NBK592401/

Potter, P., Perry, A., Stockert, P., & Hall, A. (2022). *Fundamentals of nursing* (11th ed.). Elsevier.

Rathod, M., Ross, H., & Franklin, D. (2022). Improving the accuracy and equity of pulse oximeters: Collaborative recommendations. *Journal of the American College of Cardiology, 1*(4). https://doi.org/10.1016/j.jacadv.2022.100118

Sapra, A., Malik, A., & Bhandari, P. (2023). Vital sign assessment. *StatPearls.* https://www.ncbi.nlm.nih.gov/books/NBK553213/

Whelton, P., Carey, R., Aronow, W., Casey, D., Collins, K., Dennison Himmelfarb, C., DePalma, S., Gidding, S., Jamerson, K., Jones, D., MacLaughlin, E., Muntner, P., Ovbiagele, B., Smith, S. C., Spencer, C. C., Stafford, R., Taler, S., Thomas, R., Williams, K., Williamson, J., & Wright, J. (2018). 2017 ACC/AHA/AAPA/ABC/ACPM/AGS/APhA/ASH/ASPC/NMA/PCNA guideline for the prevention, detection, evaluation, and management of high blood pressure in adults: A report of the American College of Cardiology/American Heart Association Task Force on Clinical Practice Guidelines. *Hypertension, 71*(6), e13–e115. https://www.ahajournals.org/doi/epub/10.1161/HYP.0000000000000065

CHAPTER 6

Assessing Mental Status

This chapter focuses on the components of the mental status examination, including how to assess each category and the differentiation between normal and potentially abnormal findings.

Observation

The mental status exam begins with observation—the elements that are assessed prior to an interaction with a patient—and then moves inward to more detailed observations elicited during the interview.

The elements of the mental status exam are a collection of data points to assess for a change in functioning at a *snapshot in time*. The elements of the exam are identified in Table 6.1 with examples of findings within normal limits (typical) and the accompanying atypical findings. The findings are inferred and used to either corroborate or contradict other findings in a mental health assessment.

TABLE 6.1 Documentation of Observed Appearance

Element	Findings Within Normal Limits	Atypical Findings
Appearance (observation of the patient's age, dress, grooming, and hygiene)	Appears as stated age, dressed appropriately for the weather, clean, well groomed, good hygiene	Looks younger or older than stated age, not appropriately dressed for the weather, unkempt, disheveled, poor hygiene, malodorous, or poor dentition
Demeanor and relatedness (observation of the patient's ability to engage in the interview and how they engage)	Cooperative, pleasant, calm Not in distress Appropriate to the situation	Uncooperative, hostile, agitated, avoidant, refusing to talk In distress Response is not consistent or congruent with the situation
Body movement (observation of whether the patient's behaviors are appropriate to the situation)	Calm	Fidgety or pacing, or they seem to be in slow motion In distress Unusual movements at baseline, particularly since many psychiatric medications can cause unusual movements

Behavior

The patient interview commences with deeper observations of the patient's presentation, starting with speech, affect, mood, eye contact, and level of consciousness (see Table 6.2).

Speech and fluency are evaluated passively throughout the assessment with observation of language skills and articulation. Tone of speech is the audible sound of speech of the patient. Rate of speech assesses the speed of words, while rhythm assesses the flow of words. Rhythm describes delays such as latency between questions and responses or spontaneous responses with appropriate length of time between questions and answers.

TABLE 6.2 Documentation of Observed Presentation

Element	Findings Within Normal Limits	Atypical Findings
Speech (tone, rate, and rhythm)	Tone within normal limits Rate within normal limits Rhythm within normal limits	Loud, soft, child-like, rapid, slowed, slurred, or latency
Fluency (ability to choose appropriate vocabulary and sentence structure)	Fluent	Word-finding difficulties Note: If the patient's native language is different from the language being used during the assessment, this may contribute to difficulty with vocabulary and not be indicative of altered mental status or neurocognitive disorder.
Content and coherence (ability to organize thoughts and stay on topic)	Clear, organized, and relatable	Difficult to understand or follow
Eye contact (level of consistency in looking in practitioner's eyes during the interaction, as appropriate to patient's culture)	Maintains appropriate eye contact	Minimal, avoidant, intense, poor, or no eye contact
Level of consciousness (ability to stay alert, awake, and aware while appropriately responding to stimuli such as questions and conversations)	Alert and aware Energetic or animated	Confused Sleepy, sluggish (lethargic) Apathetic (lacking interest)
Affect (emotional expression during the interview that assesses range and appropriateness to the situation)	Congruent (appropriate to situation) Full range of affect	Incongruent (not appropriate to situation) Overly excitable Flat or unchanged
Mood (subjective description of patient when asked, "How are you feeling today?"; assessed for appropriateness)	"Happy" "Worried" "Sad, depressed" "Angry"	

Thought Process

Thought process assesses the way in which a patient thinks and whether the patient *makes sense*. It is the organization of thoughts that is being assessed (see Table 6.3).

TABLE 6.3 Documentation of Observed Thought Process

Element	Findings Within Normal Limits	Atypical Findings
Thought process	Logical, organized, goal-directed (clear connection between what is being said and how it is being said)	Disorganized (illogical)
		Thought blocking (long pauses)
		Circumstantial (thoughts go off on a tangent, then return to original point)
		Tangential (thoughts go off on a tangent and don't return to the original topic)

Thought Content

The thought content section of the mental status exam assesses for risk and safety as well as the subject matter of the patient's thoughts called perceptions—specifically, impairment in perception, which is the presence of difficulty differentiating between what is reality and what might be a disturbance in reality, such as delusions, illusions, or hallucinations.

Patients may experience feelings of guilt, helplessness, or worthlessness that can contribute to the risk for physical harm to themselves or others. Many variables can contribute to this experience, such as grief and loss, new health issues, change to employment status, or change in relationship status. It is important to ask about safety and be comfortable with asking affirmative questions that are closed-ended (yes or no responses) to clarify safety concerns. It sometimes feels uncomfortable to ask about risk and safety due to your own discomfort with the information being shared by the patient. The myth is that if you ask the question, the question may spark an idea in the patient. This belief is false. Asking the question does not plant ideas in a patient's mind. It is important to note that not all patients diagnosed with depression experience suicidal ideation, and not all patients who experience suicidal ideation are diagnosed with depression. Although the experience of suicidal ideation is debilitating, its disclosure often indicates the patient's willingness to receive help. If information is disclosed in an interaction, promptly inform a mental health professional, or connect the patient with the nearest available resource for further assessment and evaluation.

Questions to elicit safety and risk are generalized to elicit the presence of thoughts of self-harm, thoughts of harm to others, and thoughts about dying, with further clarification about plans, means, and intent asked more specifically.

Perceptions

Questions about perceptual experiences such as hallucinations, paranoia, or sensory distortions assess a patient's capacity to maintain awareness of reality. Perceptions are considered the *subject matter* of the patient's thoughts. A common way to elicit perceptions is through direct questions to obtain information:

Paranoia: Are you feeling watched or controlled?

Delusions (fixed beliefs not based in reality): Are you having delusions? If so, about what?

Phobias: Are you afraid of any specific things, places, or experiences?

Hallucinations (can be experienced through any of the five senses): Do you hear things that other people may not hear? Do you see things that other people may not see? Do you smell things that are not present? Do you ever feel sensations on your body without anyone or anything present to cause them? Do you ever taste something that is not being eaten?

Observe the patient's affect during their responses. Is the thought content consistent with their affect? Does the patient appear distressed or relaxed?

Cognition

The patient interaction continues to unfold with more data collection in the assessment. *Cognition* refers to a patient's mental processes relating to gathering and understanding information. The elements of assessment in the cognition section of the mental status exam involve memory, problem-solving, logic, reasoning, and attention.

Memory

Memory is discretely assessed via recent (short-term) memory and remote (long-term) memory.

An example of a way to elicit short-term memory is to give three items of different categories at a certain point during the interview and allow the interview to progress for five to seven minutes, then ask for the patient to recall the items asked previously. Example: book, flower, and train; or numbers such as 2, 195, and 78.

Logic, Reasoning, and Attention

This is the section of the mental status exam where attention is assessed. The use of simple mathematical problems or spelling can ascertain important information. Methods of collecting data include asking a patient to count by sevens or spell the word "world" backwards. Awareness of person, place, time, and situation assesses for orientation. General information can also be requested on current affairs to assess the patient's knowledge base. Additionally, questions about how to resolve an issue can be utilized to assess problem-solving capacity. Be sure to ask questions unique to the patient's lifestyle, such as asking a social media manager how to post content in order of steps to assess the patient based on experience and interest. Visual and spatial ability can be assessed by asking the patient to draw a face on a clock and set the hands to a particular time.

Problem-solving and attention span questions assess the patient's capacity to think about the most appropriate way to manage a situation and the ability to stay present and focused for the assessment.

Insight and Judgment

Insight is an internalized process and is defined as a patient's understanding of their impairment and ability to function. Documentation of insight is usually described as limited, poor, or fair and—if there is previous comparison available—worsening versus improving.

Judgment is an externalized behavior and defined as a patient's ability to understand and make good decisions. Judgment is assessed by asking a patient what they would do in specific scenarios. Like insight, judgment is also rated as poor, limited, fair, or—if there is a previous evaluation to compare to—worsening versus improving (see Table 6.4).

TABLE 6.4 Documentation of Insight and Judgment

Element	Findings Within Normal Limits	Atypical Findings
Insight (internal understanding of one's impairment or ability to function)	Fair, good, or improving	Limited, poor, or worsening
Judgment (ability to understand and make good decisions)	Fair, good, or improving	Limited, poor, or worsening

When to introduce this chapter: This chapter would be appropriate to introduce as part of a comprehensive H&P as well as part of a neurological exam.

Class Discussion Prompts

What are some "red flags" within the mental status exam that would prompt the nurse to assess further?

What abnormal findings would prompt the nurse to initiate additional safety precautions and/or to notify the provider?

What might a mental status exam look like for patients with various psychiatric illnesses (e.g., major depressive disorder, generalized anxiety disorder, schizophrenia, Alzheimer's disease, mania, etc.)?

What type(s) of patient presentation(s) and/or chief complaints would prompt the nurse to perform a full mental status exam versus a brief one?

Class Activity

Have the students complete mental status exams on each other in groups of two. Students should take turns being the "patient" and should answer the mental status questions and challenges as if they were a person with a specific psychiatric disorder such as the ones listed above.

The interviewing student will then practice writing up the results of the mental status exam to practice documentation and make a list of 1) further assessments to perform and 2) potential mental health diagnoses the patient may have. Then have students switch roles.

Discuss with the class.

CHAPTER 7

Assessment Considerations for the Geriatric Patient

This chapter focuses on special considerations for geriatric assessment and highlights common variations in presentation that develop as a normal part of the aging process. The case involves a 72-year-old male who has received limited healthcare. He is currently residing with his son, who has concerns for his father's safety and mental status. The case reviews common screening techniques for fall risk, hypertension, and general wellness. It includes pertinent points for patient education and directed nursing care, including the process of medication reconciliation.

When to introduce this chapter: This chapter would be appropriate for assessment techniques for the elderly patient, including normal variations of aging, screening for and management of fall risk, and the concepts of polypharmacy and the nurse's role in pharmacological risk reduction.

Class Discussion Prompts

What is a normal variant of aging that may impair a patient's capability for self-care?

What is polypharmacy? Why are elderly patients more at risk for polypharmacy? What nursing actions can help prevent polypharmacy and its potential associated negative outcomes?

Class Activity

Have the students walk through their homes to identify potential fall risks. Students will then draft a remediation plan to improve the safety profile of their home.

CHAPTER 8

Assessment Considerations for the Pediatric Patient

This chapter reviews the case of Susie Lynn, a healthy 6-year-old female who presents for a school physical. The case reviews a pediatric physical exam: vaccination scheduling (including HPV vaccination), height and weight measurement, growth percentile chart graphing (see Figure 8.1), and family education on wellness in the pediatric patient.

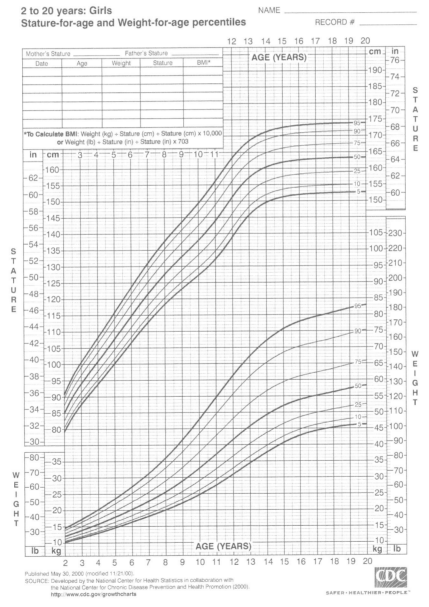

FIGURE 8.1 CDC growth reference chart (CDC, 2017).

When to introduce this chapter: This chapter is appropriately paired with lectures on pediatric development and milestones. It offers robust explanation of vaccination scheduling, thus serving as a valuable resource when reviewing vaccination administration recommendations.

Class Discussion Prompts

What are some techniques you might employ to actively engage the pediatric patient during the subjective section of their exam? How might your technique change based on the age of the child?

Pediatric obesity is a global health problem that greatly impacts the United States. What patient education is valuable for the pediatric patient and their caregivers when addressing a child with an abnormally high BMI? Since this can be a sensitive subject, what therapeutic communication techniques might be helpful to share information without seeming judgmental?

Class Activity

Break students into small groups and assign each a body system. Particular to that assigned system, instruct the students to list five ways their examination techniques would differ between the pediatric patient and the adult patient. This may be physical differences or differences in technique. For example: For an adult patient you would pull the ear lobe up and back, and for a child, you would pull the ear lobe down and out to facilitate otoscopic examination.

Groups will then share their lists with the class and discuss.

CHAPTER 9
Neurological Anomalies

This chapter follows the case of Mr. Smith, a 67-year-old male patient who sustains a cerebral vascular accident. Information includes abnormal vital signs that may be evident in a patient with a neurological event, identification of predisposing factors for stroke, basics of neurological assessment and recognition of symptoms that may be associated with impaired neurological status, and the assessment and safety of patients with seizure activity.

When to introduce this chapter: This chapter is appropriate when introducing content on neurological assessment. It may also be useful when addressing considerations for patients with seizure disorders or discussing the management of a patient with cardiovascular disease.

Class Discussion Prompts

In the instance that you are tasked with assessing a nonverbal patient, what are some assessment techniques that you might use to determine factors such as cognition or pain level?

The chapter includes the following tables and figures to aid students in answering these questions.

TABLE 9.1 Levels of Consciousness

Level of Consciousness	Description
Conscious	Normal; responds appropriately to questions of orientation
Confused	Impaired thinking and responses; disordered attention along with diminished speed, clarity, and coherence of thought (Adams et al., 1997)
Delirious	Disoriented; restlessness, hallucinations, sometimes delusions; disturbance in attention (reduced ability to direct, focus, sustain, and shift attention) and awareness (American Psychiatric Association, 2013)
Somnolent	Sleepy; excessive drowsiness, difficult to arouse, responds to stimuli in a disorganized manner
Obtunded	Decreased alertness; slowed psychomotor responses
Stuporous	Sleep-like state (not unconscious); little/no spontaneous activity; response with grimace or withdrawal from painful stimuli
Comatose	Cannot be aroused; nonresponsive to verbal or painful stimuli

(Porth, 2007)

Glasgow Coma Scale		
Response	**Scale**	**Score**
Eye Opening Response	Eyes open spontaneously	4 Points
	Eyes open to verbal command, speech, or shout	3 Points
	Eyes open to pain (not applied to face)	2 Points
	No eye opening	1 Point
Verbal Response	Oriented	5 Points
	Confused conversation, but able to answer questions	4 Points
	Inappropriate responses, words discernible	3 Points
	Incomprehensible sounds or speech	2 Points
	No verbal response	1 Point
Motor Response	Obeys commands for movement	6 Points
	Purposeful movement to painful stimulus	5 Points
	Withdraws from pain	4 Points
	Abnormal (spastic) flexion, decorticate posture	3 Points
	Extensor (rigid) response, decerebrate posture	2 Points
	No motor response	1 Point

Minor Brain Injury = 13-15 points; **Moderate Brain Injury** = 9-12 points; **Severe Brain Injury** = 3-8 points

FIGURE 9.1 Glasgow Coma Scale scoring.

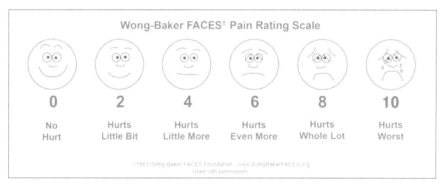

FIGURE 9.2 Wong-Baker FACES Scale.

TABLE 9.2 Cranial Nerves

Number	Name	Function
I	Olfactory	Smell
II	Optic	Sight
III	Oculomotor	Moves eye, pupillary movement
IV	Trochlear	Moves eye
V	Trigeminal	Facial sensation
VI	Abducens	Moves eye
VII	Facial	Facial movement, salivation
VIII	Vestibulocochlear	Hearing, balance
IX	Glossopharyngeal	Taste, swallow

Number	Name	Function
X	Vagus	Heart rate, digestion
XI	Accessory	Moves head
XII	Hypoglossal	Moves tongue

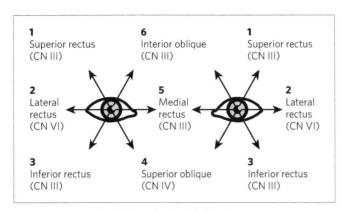

FIGURE 9.3 Cardinal fields of gaze.

Class Activity

Break students into 12 groups. Open a shared document (such as Google Docs) and invite all students to participate. Assign each of the 12 groups a cranial nerve. In the document, each group will add information on the function of their assigned cranial nerve, as well as assessment methods particular to that nerve. Once each group has contributed, students will have a collaborative document that details the function and assessment of each cranial nerve to use as a study reference.

Afterward, ask each group to present their findings.

REFERENCES

Adams, R. D., Victor M., & Ropper, A. H. (1997). Delirium and other acute confusional states. In R. D. Adams, M. Victor, & A. H. Ropper (Eds)., *Principles of neurology* (6th ed., pp. 431–443). McGraw Hill.

American Psychiatric Association. (2013). *Diagnostic and statistical manual of mental disorders* (5th ed.). Author.

Porth, C. (2007). *Essentials of pathophysiology: Concepts of altered health states*. Lippincott Williams & Wilkins.

Wong-Baker FACES Foundation. (2016). *Faces of pain care*. https://wongbakerfaces.org/

CHAPTER 10

Cardiovascular and Vascular Anomalies

Chapter 10 reviews the case of Mr. Jones, a 60-year-old male who sustains a myocardial infarction (MI). It reviews pertinent cardiac risk factors and findings associated with MI. The chapter provides a detailed description of the cardiac exam, including assessment of the precordium, cardiac auscultatory techniques, assessment of murmurs, and basic ECG findings. The case goes on to describe the procedure of cardiac catheterization and postsurgical monitoring that progresses to congestive heart failure.

Signs and Symptoms of Myocardial Infarction in Males vs. Females

Signs and symptoms of MI might include (Heart.org, 2022):

- Chest discomfort usually described as crushing, squeezing, or fullness in the center or left side of the chest
- Pain radiating into one or both arms, the jaw, or the back
- Shortness of breath
- Nausea, vomiting, or diaphoresis (sweating)
- Lightheadedness

These symptoms will vary in presentation and intensity from one patient to the next. Some patients suffering from MI appear to be in acute distress, as is the case with Mr. Jones, while others are unaware they are experiencing an MI at all, which occurs during a silent MI (FamilyDoctor.org, 2023).

Historically, men have received more medical referrals and care for the prevention and treatment of coronary heart disease, the predisposing condition to MI development. In more recent years, there has been a movement to increase education and awareness of women's risk for developing MI. When discussing heart attack risk with female patients, the potential for atypical MI presentation is critical. Women are more likely to experience vague or mild symptoms including (Heart.org, 2022):

- Burning sensation in their upper abdomen
- Back pain
- Aching jaw
- Lightheadedness
- Upset stomach
- Sweating

Many times, these symptoms are attributed to other conditions like indigestion. Heart attacks tend to be more severe in women. In the first year after an MI, women are 50% more likely than men to die from coronary disease or complications (Texas Heart Institute, n.d.).

When to introduce this chapter: This chapter will be helpful when introducing concepts of cardiac assessment and ECG interpretation.

Class Discussion Prompts

MI is more likely to occur undetected in female patients. Why is this? What are some of the major differences between how male and female patients might experience symptoms of MI?

Formulate three subjective questions that would provide more information regarding a patient's risk for developing coronary artery disease.

Class Activity

Preparation: Although venous and arterial disease are classified as peripheral vascular disorders, their implications and presenting symptoms are vastly different. Prepare a list of objective and subjective findings of peripheral vascular disease.

Activity: Break students into small groups, and present each with the list of objective and subjective findings of peripheral vascular disease. Ask them to determine which findings are associated with venous peripheral vascular disease and which are associated with arterial peripheral vascular disease.

Groups should share their responses with the class and discuss.

REFERENCES

FamilyDoctor.org. (2023). *Silent heart attacks.* https://familydoctor.org/condition/silent-heart-attacks/

Heart.org. (2022). *Heart attack symptoms in women.* https://www.heart.org/en/health-topics/heart-attack/warning-signs-of-a-heart-attack/heart-attack-symptoms-in-women

Texas Heart Institute. (n.d.). *Women and heart disease.* https://www.texasheart.org/heart-health/heart-information-center/topics/women-and-heart-disease/

CHAPTER 11

Respiratory Anomalies

Chapter 11 reviews the case of Mrs. Brown, a 62-year-old African-American woman with a history of smoking who is diagnosed with chronic obstructive pulmonary disorder (COPD). The properties of the respiratory assessment are reviewed during this case, including techniques of auscultation and percussion and indications for imaging.

Signs and Symptoms of Advanced Lung Disease

Subjective data include:

- Shortness of breath on exertion for past 18 months
- Fatigue during usual activities, requiring assistance
- Chest tightness
- Asthma inhaler unhelpful and barely used
- Cough present for approximately nine weeks
- 25.5 pack year history
- Two to three times weekly exposure to unfiltered cigar smoke

Objective data include:

- Vital signs, especially her respiratory rate (RR), which is notably high
- Diagnosed with acute bronchitis 3x in past 12 months (verified by EHR, so objective in this case because it can be confirmed)
- Cyanosis of nailbeds
- Productive cough (objective here because witnessed by the RN during assessment)
- Tripod position
- Pallor in face
- Wheezes heard bilaterally on auscultation

When to introduce this chapter: The chapter will be useful when introducing concepts of a basic respiratory assessment and findings associated with chronic respiratory conditions such as COPD and emphysema.

Class Discussion Prompts

Emphysema and chronic bronchitis are both classified as chronic obstructive pulmonary diseases even though the pathology of each is very different. What are the differences between the pathophysiology of the two conditions, and how do those differences manifest during the physical assessment?

Preparation: Create a vignette of a patient who currently smokes.

Activity: Smoking cessation is most successful with strong patient support from medical providers. Provide the students with the vignette of a patient who currently smokes and ask them to develop a resource plan for the hypothetical patient.

CHAPTER 12

Gastroenterological Anomalies

This chapter follows the case of Mrs. Johnson, a 52-year-old female patient diagnosed with cirrhosis. Content includes basic liver functionality, along with subjective and objective findings commonly found in the patient with liver disease.

Physical Assessment of the Abdomen

When performing a physical assessment of the abdomen (see Figure 12.1), the patient should first be asked to lie in a supine position, with arms resting to either side of the body. This position prevents tightening of the abdominal muscles (Ignatavicius & Workman, 2016). A thorough assessment of the abdomen includes inspection, auscultation, percussion, and palpation.

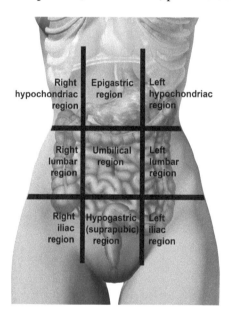

FIGURE 12.1 The nine regions of the abdomen.

The nurse first **inspects** the abdomen for overall symmetry/asymmetry and presence of discoloration, abdominal distention, and pulsations.

Next, the nurse **auscultates** all four quadrants of the abdomen with the diaphragm of a stethoscope. This should always be done prior to percussion or palpation, as the latter two assessment techniques may alter sounds (Hinkle & Cheever, 2018). The characterization of bowel sounds should be noted as normal, hypoactive, hyperactive, or absent (see Table 12.1). Bruits may be auscultated with the bell of a stethoscope. A bruit heard over the aorta may indicate the presence of an aortic aneurysm.

The nurse next **percusses** the abdomen to estimate the size of solid organs, such as the liver or spleen, and to determine the presence of fluid, air, and masses. Unless a bruit is heard, all four quadrants should be percussed and the character of sound documented (see Table 12.2; Jarvis, 2012).

Lastly, the nurse **palpates** the abdomen using light palpation to assess for tenderness and deep palpation to assess for masses (Jarvis, 2012).

TABLE 12.1 Bowel Sounds

Bowel Sound	Qualities	Possible Causes
Normal	Relatively high-pitched and irregular 5–35 sounds occurring every minute or one sound every 5–15 seconds	Normally functioning intestines
Hypoactive	Softer and widespread sounds Less than 5 sounds per minute or one occurring every 20 to 30 seconds or longer	Postoperative after general anesthesia Paralytic ileus Peritonitis Decreased bowel motility Late intestinal obstruction
Absent	Absence of intestinal motility No sounds heard for 5 minutes	Peritonitis Paralytic ileus (late finding) Perforation Mesenteric ischemia
Hyperactive	Loud and frequent, with 35 or more sounds per minute	Diarrhea Peritonitis Intestinal obstruction (early finding) Gastroenteritis Anxiety
Bruit	"Whooshing" sound over the abdominal aorta, renal arteries, and/or iliac arteries	Abdominal aortic aneurysm Renal artery stenosis

(Jarvis, 2012)

TABLE 12.2 Percussion Sounds

Sound	Intensity	Pitch	Quality	Duration	Common Locations
Resonance	Moderately loud	Low	Clear, hollow	Moderate	Over normal lung tissue
Hyper-resonance	Very loud	Very low	Booming	Long	Emphysematous lung
Tympany	Loud	High	Musical and drum-like	Longest	Enclosed air-filled space (e.g., stomach, intestines, puffed-out cheek)
Dullness	Soft	High	Muffled thud	Short	Dense organ (e.g., liver or spleen)
Flatness	Soft	High	Flat, absolute dullness	Very short	Areas with no air present (e.g., muscle, bone)

When to introduce this chapter: This chapter is useful when introduced with elements of gastroenterological assessment. It can also be useful in highlighting risks associated with alcoholism or the identification of chronic liver disease.

Class Discussion Prompts

Jaundice is the yellow discoloration of the skin that is commonly associated with liver disease. Why does this yellow discoloration occur? What are other symptoms of chronic liver disease?

Class Activity

Preparation: Write out the name of each major abdominal organ (see Figure 12.2) and toss it in a hat.

Activity: Break the class into groups and have each group pull the name of an organ. They are responsible for describing the function of that organ, providing a description of the pain pattern, and describing any specific assessment techniques (e.g., appendix and rebound tenderness).

When it is their turn to present, each group should identify the location of the organ, along with their assessment findings.

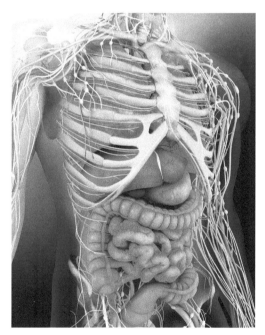

FIGURE 12.2 View of the gastrointestinal organs in relation to the skeleton.

REFERENCES

Hinkle, J. L., & Cheever, K. H. (2018). *Brunner and Suddarth's textbook of medical-surgical nursing, Volume 2* (14th ed.). Wolters Kluwer.

Ignatavicius, D. D., & Workman, M. L. (2016). *Medical-surgical nursing: Patient-centered collaborative care* (8th ed.). Elsevier.

Jarvis, C. (2012). *Physical examination and health assessment* (6th ed.). Saunders.

CHAPTER 13

Genitourinary and Sexual Health

This chapter reviews the case of Abigail, a 17-year-old female who presents with abdominal pain. The case goes on to review basic female reproductive anatomy, presentation of a patient with a urinary tract infection, screening for sexually transmitted infections, and pregnancy. A unique quality of this case is its explanation of how to approach conversations with adolescent patients accompanied by parents or caregivers.

When to introduce this chapter: This dynamic case is appropriately introduced with topics such as adolescent health, assessment of urinary tract infection, pregnancy, sexually transmitted infections, or abdominal pain.

Class Discussion Prompts

How would you approach a situation where an adolescent patient is accompanied by a parent or adult?

What are the legal implications?

How does the presence of a caregiver potentially influence your examination (positively and negatively)?

Class Activity

The patient in this case is discovered to be pregnant. Have students work together to identify three key teaching points for the expectant mother (e.g., avoiding soft cheeses and raw fish).

CHAPTER 14

Dermatological Anomalies

This case begins with Makayla, a 61-year-old female patient presenting for a routine physical examination. The interviewing nurse identifies a number of risk factors for skin cancer during the subjective portion of the exam, which ultimately leads to the identification of a suspicious lesion during the objective examination. The chapter goes into detail regarding the risk factors for developing cancer, descriptions of common skin lesions, and expected "normal" variants of aging.

Skin Cancer Risk Factors

- **Ultraviolet (UV) light exposure:** UV rays originate from the sun. Without adequate protection, they have the capability to damage skin cell DNA, causing abnormal growth, as is the case in skin cancer.

- **Presence of atypical moles:** Moles, known as *nevi,* are a normal, nonthreatening occurrence; however, if a person has more moles, they may be more likely to develop melanoma over the course of their life.

- **Fair skin:** People with white skin are at the greatest risk of developing skin cancer. Fair-skinned people, especially those with red or blonde hair, green or blue eyes, freckling, or those who sunburn easily, are at the greatest risk. However, individuals of any skin tone can potentially develop skin cancer.

- **Family history:** If a first-degree relative (a parent, sibling, or child) has had melanoma, the risk of developing the disease is higher. In fact, about 10% of patients diagnosed with melanoma have a family history of the disease.

- **Personal history of skin cancer:** Someone who has already had a diagnosis of skin cancer is at an increased risk of developing a subsequent lesion.

- **Weakened immune system:** Patients with weak immune systems are more likely to develop skin cancer. Conditions that may weaken the immune system include HIV or autoimmune diseases.

- **Advanced age:** Skin cancer can occur at any age; however, the risk increases with age.

- **Gender:** The risk is higher for women before the age of 50, but after age 50, the risk is higher in men.

Sun Safety

According to the Centers for Disease Control and Prevention (CDC), the sun's UV rays can damage the skin in as little as 15 minutes (CDC, 2023). Some ways to prevent damage from UV rays include finding shade, wearing protective clothing and hats, and wearing sunscreen. Sunscreen is rated according to its sun protection factor (SPF). A minimum SPF of 15 is recommended; the higher the SPF, the more protection the product provides from the sun. Patients must be instructed to reapply the product per manufacturer recommendations or after swimming or sweating. Sunscreen expires, like most other health and beauty products, and may not be as potent if the product has expired. Although most sun care products have a shelf life of three years, exposure to heat can damage them (CDC, 2023).

Pertinent patient teaching points should include:

1. Use of sunscreen and how to protect the skin from UV exposure
2. Recommendations for annual skin checks by a licensed dermatological provider
3. Frequent self-evaluation of skin integrity for early identification of suspicious lesions
4. How to use the ABCDE screening for self-skin checks
5. The different types of skin cancer
6. Common risk factors

The ABCDE Mnemonic for Assessing Skin Lesions

The ABCDE mnemonic stands for:

A: Asymmetry—If you were to fold the lesion in half, would the edges match? If not, the lesion is said to be asymmetrical. Asymmetry is concerning for malignancy.

B: Border—The border should appear smooth and consistent. Rough, irregular borders would be worrisome.

C: Color—Is the color of the lesion consistent throughout? If the coloration is inconsistent or contains different pigments, it would be considered suspicious.

D: Diameter—Is the lesion greater than 6 mm?

E: Elevation, enlargement, or evolution—Is the lesion raised? Or has the lesion enlarged or evolved? Change or growth may be a sign of malignancy (Duarte et al., 2021).

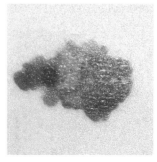

Review Figure 14.1 and apply what you know about ABCDE screening. This is an example of melanoma; you can recognize the asymmetric appearance, irregular border, and inconsistent coloration. Based on these findings, this patient would require a referral for further evaluation of the lesion.

FIGURE 14.1 Skin cancer.

When to introduce this chapter: This chapter is a natural supplement to content related to dermatological assessment. It also has a place in the discussion of normal variants of aging, with its robust description of common variants in the appearance and function of the skin in the older adult.

Class Discussion Prompts

What education can the nurse provide to the patient regarding sun safety?

What are some common misconceptions about skin cancer, and how can the nurse influence a positive change in self-care practices?

Class Activity

Preparation: Using an automatic bingo card generator (there are many available for free online), develop bingo cards using the names of primary and secondary skin lesions (e.g., papule, macule, etc.; see Table 14.1).

Activity: Each student receives a bingo card, and the instructor acts as the caller. Instead of calling the names of the terms when drawn, the instructor will only provide students with an unlabeled picture *or* description of the lesion. Students will have to rely on their integumentary vocabulary to match the photos or descriptions to the vocabulary on their bingo cards. When students get five in a row, they can call out "Bingo!" and read back the matching terms.

TABLE 14.1 Primary Skin Lesions

Lesion	Description	Example
Macule	Flat, circumscribed, less than 1 cm	Freckle, small nevus
Papule	Solid, elevated, circumscribed, less than 1 cm	Wart
Vesicle	Fluid-filled blister up to 1 cm	Chicken pox, poison ivy
Bulla	Fluid-filled blister larger than 1 cm	Blister
Patch	Flat, circumscribed, greater than 1 cm	Café au lait spot
Cyst	Encapsulated, fluid-filled cavity	Cystic acne
Wheal	Superficial, raised, transient, erythematous	Mosquito bite, urticaria

(Jarvis, 2016)

REFERENCES

Centers for Disease Control and Prevention. (2023). *Sun safety.* https://www.cdc.gov/cancer/skin/basic_info/sun-safety.htm

Duarte, A. F., Sousa-Pinto, B., Azevedo, L. F., Barros, A. M., Puig, S., Malvehy, J., Haneke, E., & Correia, O. (2021). Clinical ABCDE rule for early melanoma detection. *European Journal of Dermatology, 31*(6), 771–778.

Jarvis, C. (2016). *Physical examination & health assessment* (7th ed.). Elsevier.

CHAPTER 15

Head and Neck Anomalies

This chapter involves Jordan, a 32-year-old female who presents to an outpatient clinic with complaints consistent with an acute sinus infection. The nurse proceeds to perform an examination of the ears, nose, and throat. Details of the examination technique, along with pertinent terminology, are introduced throughout the case. During her exam, the nurse discovers an enlarged thyroid gland, and the case further develops to address a new diagnosis of hypothyroidism.

Hypothyroidism refers to a state of underactive thyroid function; *hyperthyroidism,* on the other hand, is an overactive thyroid. See Table 15.1.

TABLE 15.1 Thyroid Dysfunction

Hypothyroidism	Hyperthyroidism
Dry hair	Hair loss
Puffy face	Bulging eyes
Slow heartbeat	Sweating
Weight gain	Elevated heartbeat
Constipation	Weight loss
Brittle nails	Sleep disturbances
Joint pain/muscle aches	Heat intolerance
Cold intolerance	Infertility
Depressed mood	Irritability
Dry skin	Muscle fatigue
Fatigue	Anxiety
Memory loss	
Heavy menstruation	

(Mayo Clinic, 2022)

When to introduce this chapter: This chapter can be introduced with content regarding examination techniques of the head and neck including the ears, nose, and throat. It is equally relevant when reviewing the assessment of thyroid disorders.

Class Discussion Prompts

What is the difference between hypothyroidism and hyperthyroidism?

What are the differences in the subjective and objective presentation of each condition?

Class Activity

Preparation: Select images of a normal tympanic membrane, a sclerosed membrane, and a case of otitis media (see Figure 15.1 for structures of the ear).

Activity: Display one image at a time for the students to evaluate and describe—encourage them to identify landmarks. Encourage the use of correct terminology when describing what they see (e.g., instead of saying "red" they should say "erythematous"). They can compete either as a class or in small groups.

This activity can also be repeated with images of the eye or throat.

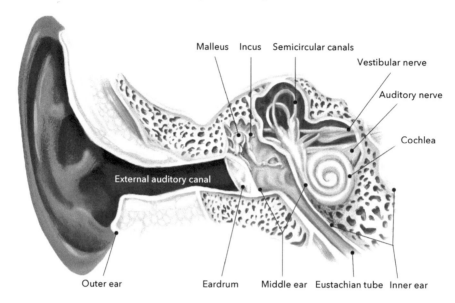

FIGURE 15.1 Structures of the ear.

REFERENCE

Mayo Clinic. (2022). *Hyperthyroidism (overactive thyroid)*. https://www.mayoclinic.org/diseases-conditions/hyperthyroidism/symptoms-causes/syc-20373659

CHAPTER 16

Assessment of the Transgender Patient

This chapter follows the case of Max, a 34-year-old transgender male who is establishing care with a new primary care provider. Max reveals during his interview that he is the victim of intimate partner violence (IPV). The chapter reviews appropriate LGBTQIA+ terminology, including gender identities and pronouns. The chapter explores hormone therapies and associated risks, as well as anticipated assessment findings.

The chapter also includes a review of the types of IPV and an IPV risk assessment.

LGBTQIA+ Terminology and Inclusion Resources

Facilitators may want to provide resources such as:

- Fenway Institute. (2020). *LGBTQIA+ glossary of terms for health care teams*. https://www.lgbtqiahealtheducation.org/publication/lgbtqia-glossary-of-terms-for-health-care-teams/

- GLAAD. (2018). *GLAAD media reference guide* (11th ed.). https://glaad.org/reference/trans-terms/

- Human Rights Campaign. (n.d.). *Sexual orientation and gender identity definitions*. https://www.hrc.org/resources/sexual-orientation-and-gender-identity-terminology-and-definitions

- National Center for Transgender Equality. (2023). *Understanding non-binary people: How to be respectful and supportive*. https://transequality.org/issues/resources/understanding-non-binary-people-how-to-be-respectful-and-supportive

- Trans Student Educational Resources. (2019). *Gender pronouns*. http://www.transstudent.org/pronouns101

- University of California, San Francisco. (2016). *Transgender care: Terminology and definitions*. https://transcare.ucsf.edu/guidelines/terminology

- University of Wisconsin, Milwaukee. (2019). *Gender pronouns*. https://uwm.edu/lgbtrc/support/gender-pronouns/

When to introduce this chapter: This chapter will supplement content on LGBTQ populations, social inclusion, and social justice. Additionally, its focus on IPV makes it applicable to curricula on domestic violence and abuse.

Class Discussion Prompts

Nurses are mandatory reporters of confirmed or suspected abuse in at-risk populations. What does this mean? How would you approach a situation where you suspected abuse?

Class Activity

This activity focuses more on class discussion to increase social awareness and acceptance. Using Tables 16.1 and 16.2, guide students in a conversation on using inclusive language. Give examples of what is and what is not considered to be inclusive language.

Ask for student input on what constitutes an "inclusive environment" and how the nurse can influence social inclusion for a diverse patient population.

TABLE 16.1 Culturally Sensitive Gender-Identity and Sexual-Orientation Terminology

Sexual Orientation	Gender Identity	Nonbinary Gender
Straight	Cisgender	Agender
Gay	Transgender male	Androgyne
Lesbian	Transgender female	Bigender
Bisexual	Gender neutral	Nonbinary
Pansexual	Two-spirit	Queer
Queer		Gender-fluid
Asexual		Gender variant
		Pangender
		Third gender

TABLE 16.2 Gender Pronouns or Gender-Neutral Pronouns

Subjective	Objective	Possessive
He	Him	His
She	Her	Hers
They	Them	Theirs
Ze/Zi	Zer/Zir	Zers/Zirs

Practice Test

The practice tests offer a collection of NCLEX-style questions including NextGen formatted items. The questions are focused on health assessment and general wellness and incorporate content from each case study in the text.

1. When assessing a patient's level of consciousness using the Glasgow Coma Scale (GCS), the nurse interprets a score of 4 as:

   A) Normal function
   B) Minor brain injury
   C) Moderate brain injury
   D) Severe brain injury

2. At the change of shift, the nurse reads the narrative note from the previous shift. The patient is noted to have miotic pupils, meaning:

   A) Dilated
   B) Constricted
   C) Uneven
   D) Unreactive

3. A 60-year-old client recently suffered a hemorrhagic stroke. Following the stroke, his family reports changes to his affect and personality. This is most likely the result of damage to:

   A) Frontal lobe
   B) Pariteal lobe
   C) Broca's area
   D) Occipital lobe

4. The nurse is performing a focused neurological assessment for a patient with optic migraines. He proceeds to examine the patient's extraocular motion by performing the six cardinal fields of gaze test. What cranial nerves are being tested during this exam?

   A) 3, 4, 6
   B) 5, 7, 8
   C) 3, 6, 7
   D) 2, 5, 8

5. During a neurological exam, the patient is unable to correctly identify the smell of cinnamon. This may potentially indicate an issue with cranial nerve _____.

   A) 3
   B) 2
   C) 4
   D) 1

6. The nurse auscultates a new onset murmur in a 22-year-old male. The murmur occurs between S2 and the subsequent S1. This would be classified as a:

   A) Systolic murmur
   B) Diastolic murmur
   C) Benign murmur
   D) Pathological murmur

7. Which of the following statements is *true* regarding the correct stethoscope placement during cardiac auscultation?

    A) The aortic valve can be auscultated at the 2nd intercostal space at the left sternal border.

    B) Erb's point can be auscultated at the 3rd intercostal space at the left sternal border.

    C) The pulmonic valve can be auscultated at the 4th intercostal space at the right sternal border.

    D) The tricuspid valve can be auscultated at the 5th intercostal space at the midclavicular line.

8. When examining the neck, the nurse appreciates a prominent bulging of the jugular vein. This condition may indicate fluid volume overload and is known as:

    A) Carotid bruit   C) Jugular venous distention

    B) Thyroidmegaly   D) Tracheal deviation

9. You are assessing your patient diagnosed with exacerbated congestive heart failure (CHF). Which abnormal heart sound is correlated with systemic volume overload in CHF?

    A) S_3 C) Mitral click

    B) Split S_1 D) S_2

10. The nurse is documenting vital signs from morning rounds. He records the patient's pulse as "regular, 72 bpm, 3+". This means:

    A) The pulse was regular in occurrence at a rate of 72 and is bounding in strength.

    B) The pulse was irregular in occurrence at a rate of 72 and is thready in strength.

    C) The pulse was regular in occurrence at a rate of 72 and is normal in strength.

    D) The pulse was irregular in occurrence at a rate of 72 and is diminished in strength.

11. A patient with a history of hyperlipidemia and hypertension presents to his primary care provider with complaints of leg pain that occurs when walking and dissipates at rest. He is concerned because his father had a similar condition that was related to arterial blockage in the legs. This leg pain is known as:

    A) Deep vein thrombosis   C) Intermittent claudication

    B) Varicose veins   D) Terminal ischemia

12. As the nurse proceeds with an examination of the skin, hair, and nails, he notices the capillary refill to be six seconds. This is significant because:

    A) It is a normal capillary refill.

    B) This indicates brisk refill, which indicates good circulation.

    C) This indicates sluggish refill, which indicates poor circulation.

    D) This indicates brisk refill, which indicates adequate hydration.

13. A patient presents with complaints of nausea, vomiting, and diarrhea for the past three days. She has not been able to tolerate food or fluids. The nurse is concerned about the patient's hydration status. Which of the following exam techniques would indicate the patient's hydration status?

A) Capillary refill

B) Murphy's sign

C) Schamroth's sign

D) Skin turgor

14. When evaluating a skin lesion for potential malignancy, the nurse recognizes that a lesion greater than _____ in diameter is considered to be highly suspicious.

A) 6 mm

B) 5 mm

C) 4 mm

D) 3 mm

15. After performing an assessment of the skin, the nurse proceeds to document his findings. During the examination, he noticed a single, flat, hyperpigmented lesion with symmetric borders and a diameter of 5 mm. The nurse would document this lesion as a:

A) Papule

B) Macule

C) Vesicle

D) Patch

16. A nurse working in a long-term care facility is taking care of a 75-year-old female patient. The patient tells the nurse she is concerned about the dark spots she has noticed on the back of her hands. The nurse tells the patient that these spots likely represent:

A) Melanoma

B) Pediculus humanus

C) Senile purpura

D) Tinea corporis

17. Which symptoms may indicate that a patient with hypothyroidism may require an increase in their thyroid replacement medication? *(Select all that apply)*

A) Fatigue

B) Bulging eyes

C) Hair loss

D) Cold intolerance

E) Weight gain

18. While examining the left tympanic membrane, the nurse appreciates the tympanic reflection, known as the cone of light, at:

A) 3 o'clock

B) 5 o'clock

C) 7 o'clock

D) 9 o'clock

19. An 18-month old boy presents with his mother, who suspects her son has an ear infection. He had been up all night with a low-grade fever and has been tugging at his right ear lobe. When proceeding with the otoscopic exam, the nurse correctly positions the ear lobe by:

A) Pulling the helix up and back

B) Compressing the tragus

C) Pushing down on the lobule

D) Pulling the helix down and out

20. While assessing a patient's lymph nodes, the nurse notes a tender, mobile lymph node palpable directly in front of the ear. When documenting the lymphadenopathy, the nurse documents tenderness of the _____ nodes.

    A) Submental   C) Jugulodigastric
    B) Preauricular   D) Superficial cervical

21. A patient diagnosed with streptococcal pharyngitis is observed to have tonsils with patchy exudate occupying approximately 60% of the oropharyngeal width. The tonsils are graded as:

    A) 1+   C) 3+
    B) 2+   D) 4+

22. Your patient was diagnosed with acute cholecystitis. As the nurse assigned to this patient, you understand that the patient will most likely have the following symptom:

    A) Epigastric pain that is relieved with eating
    B) Epigastric pain that is aggravated with a high fat meal
    C) Left lower quadrant with rebound tenderness
    D) A negative Murphy's sign

23. You are educating a patient who has been diagnosed with cirrhosis about esophageal varices. You advise the patient to avoid the following activities, if possible: *(Select all that apply)*

    A) Consuming alcohol
    B) Vomiting
    C) Sleeping in a lateral recumbent position
    D) Eating spicy foods
    E) Excessive coughing

24. Your patient was recently admitted with acute pancreatitis. As the nurse caring for this patient, you know the patient's risk factors include all *except*:

    A) Heavy alcohol use   C) Diabetes mellitus
    B) Smoking   D) Obesity

25. A patient is admitted to the ED with complaint of pain around the umbilicus that radiates to the lower abdominal region on the right. Pain is elicited while palpating the right lower quadrant of the abdomen (about one-third the distance between the anterior superior iliac spine and the umbilicus). This is known as:

    A) Positive Murphy's sign   C) Positive McBurney's sign
    B) Positive Rovsing's sign   D) Positive Trousseau's sign

26. You are the nurse taking care of a patient that is four days post-op after an appendectomy. Which assessment finding requires further evaluation?

    A) The patient reports only tolerating clear liquids.
    B) The patient reports incisional pain.
    C) The patient reports his last bowel movement was pre-operative.
    D) A and C

27. You are providing education to a patient newly diagnosed with a duodenal ulcer. Which of the following statements indicates that reeducation may be needed?

    A) "I should eat smaller meals throughout the day instead of three large ones."
    B) "I should avoid coffee, chocolate, and fried foods."
    C) "Eating will only make my pain worse."
    D) "I should report any dark, tarry bowel movements."

28. You are caring for a patient who presented to the hospital with a temperature of 101.9°F and abdominal pain. Workup in the emergency department included sending blood samples to the lab for a variety of tests. A complete blood count revealed an elevated white blood cell count. It is suspected that your patient has diverticulitis. Which of the following statements is correct regarding diverticulitis?

    A) Oatmeal and nuts are the best foods for acute diverticulitis.
    B) Diverticulitis is usually associated with a positive Cullen's sign.
    C) Patients with diverticulitis should be encouraged to drink clear liquids.
    D) A positive Murphy's sign is indicative of diverticulitis.

29. The nurse is performing an obstetrical history and needs the date of the last menstrual period to determine the estimated date of birth using Nagel's rule. The nurse asks the patient:

    A) What was the last day of your last period?
    B) What was the heaviest day of your last menstrual period?
    C) What was the first day of your last menstrual cycle?
    D) What was the last month you had a menstrual period?

30. The patient presents with complaints of frequent urge to void, nausea and vomiting, burning during urination, chills, fever, costal vertebral angle tenderness, and pain in the lower abdomen radiating to the back. The nurse correctly suspects the following condition:

    A) Cystitis   C) Ovarian cyst
    B) Pregnancy   D) Pyelonephritis

31. During patient teaching, the nurse explains gynecological care and steps to take to prevent sexually transmitted infections (STIs). *(Select all that apply)*

    A) Limit the number of sexual partners.
    B) Get tested yearly for chlamydia and gonorrhea after 25 years of age.
    C) Use condoms consistently.
    D) Talk to your sexual partners about their history with STI.
    E) Ask your provider if STI screening is offered.

32. The patient presents to the ED and explains she is currently pregnant, has a 3-year-old child born at 39 weeks, and also lost a pregnancy in the first trimester. The nurse documents her GTPAL as:

    A) G2 T1 P1 A0 L1   C) G2 T0 P0 A1 L2
    B) G3 T1 P0 A1 L1   D) G3 T1 P1 A0 L2

33. The nurse admits a patient into labor and delivery and needs to calculate her due date. Using Nagel's rule and the date of July 20, 2023, determine her estimated date of birth.

    A) April 27, 2024   C) March 20, 2024
    B) February 23, 2024   D) May 27, 2024

34. The nurse is planning a patient education program about urinary tract infections (UTIs) across the life span. Which of the following correct statements will the nurse include in the educational discussion? *(Select all that apply)*

    A) UTIs are a very common type of infection, mostly affecting children under the age of 5 and men and women aged 70 and older.
    B) People with high blood glucose levels are especially susceptible to getting a UTI.
    C) For prevention, drink plenty of water, urinate often, keep your genital area clean, and empty your bladder before and after sex.
    D) There is conclusive evidence to using cranberry supplement products to prevent UTIs.

35. The nurse in a urology practice discusses bladder health with her many patients. Which of the following female patient statements is a reason for concern? *(Select all that apply)*

    A) "I have been doing my Kegel exercises three times a day for the past two weeks, and I still do not see any improvement."
    B) "I am drinking about 2 liters of fluid a day and urinating about 500 liters."
    C) "I don't like to sit while I void, and I find myself going to the bathroom about 14 times a day."
    D) "I wipe from front to back after using the toilet."

36. When assessing the geriatric client, the nurse correctly acknowledges which of the following as a normal variant of aging?

    A) Low-frequency hearing loss   C) Increased muscle mass
    B) Hypertrophied skin surfaces   D) Decreased metabolism

37. A 70-year-old male presents for a wellness visit. Which of the following is expected to be included as part of routine health maintenance for this patient?

    A) Prostate specific antigen (PSA)
    B) Brain magnetic resonance imaging (MRI)
    C) Cardiac stress test
    D) BRACA-1 testing

38. Which of the following physiological changes in the elderly patient is *not* considered to be a risk factor for increased fall risk?

    A) Decreased muscle strength
    B) Increased reflexes
    C) Decreased step height
    D) Increased postural sway

39. When evaluating the fall risk for a patient, which tool is used to determine the patient's likelihood of falling?

    A) Downton Fall Risk Index
    B) Hendrich II Fall Risk Model
    C) Timed Up and Go test
    D) A combined assessment approach is preferred.

40. The nurse is discussing risk factors for dementia with a patient and his caregiver. When discussing potential risk factors for the development of dementia, the nurse includes: *(Select all that apply)*

    A) Obesity
    B) Decreased HDL cholesterol
    C) Hypotension
    D) Smoking
    E) Low physical exercise

41. A nurse is caring for a patient who complains of feeling short of breath. Respiratory rate is recorded at 28 breaths per minute. Before contacting the provider, the nurse should *first*:

    A) Raise the head of the bed 45 degrees
    B) Administer 2L O2 via nasal cannula
    C) Administer CPR
    D) Check the patient's blood pressure

42. A nurse is providing discharge information for a patient with recently diagnosed asthma. Which of the following common triggers for asthma should the nurse instruct the patient to try to avoid? *(Select all that apply)*

    A) Cat and dog dander
    B) Humidified rooms
    C) Sunlight
    D) Tobacco smoke
    E) Chewing tobacco
    F) Wood burning stoves

43. An African-American patient with COPD seeks emergency care for acute respiratory distress. For patients with dark skin color, the nurse should assess for cyanosis by inspecting the:

A) Lips

C) Thorax

B) Mucous membranes

D) Nail beds

44. A pediatric patient was noted to have retractions below the xyphoid process on the upper abdomen. When recording this, the nurse labels these as:

A) Substernal retractions

C) Intercostal retractions

B) Subcostal retractions

D) Supraclavicular retractions

45. A nurse is caring for an elderly patient who is suffering from influenza. The nurse performs frequent respiratory assessments, as the nurse knows that _____ is one of the most common complications of influenza.

A) Pulmonary embolism

C) Pneumonia

B) Bacteremia

D) Guillain-Barré syndrome

46. Which of the following statements best describes sexual orientation?

A) How one identifies internally with regards to their gender

B) The romantic, physical, and psychological attraction towards another person

C) A person or persons who identify without a particular fixed gender

D) The incongruence between the sex assigned at birth and how one identifies their gender

47. Which patients should the nurse ask to identify their pronouns?

A) Patients who appear to be nonbinary

B) Patients who self-identify as transgender

C) Patients who identify as lesbian or gay

D) All patients should be asked what their self-identified pronoun is.

48. Transgender patients who take hormones such as testosterone or estrogen should be monitored for the risk of developing which of the following? *(Select all that apply)*

A) Deep vein thrombosis

D) Abnormal liver function

B) Hypertension

E) Migraines

C) Type 2 diabetes

49. Transgender persons are at higher risk for which of the following? *(Select all that apply)*

A) Double the rate of unemployment

B) Higher rates of death by suicide

C) Higher socioeconomic status

D) Acts of physical, sexual, and emotional harassment

E) Substance abuse

50. When caring for a transgender patient, which of the following would be appropriate for the nurse to consider? *(Select all that apply)*

A) Continuity of care by the same nurses as much as possible
B) Educating all caregivers on the appropriate and sensitive care of the transgender patient
C) Asking the patient to teach them about what it is like to be transgender
D) Minimizing the patient's visitors during their hospitalization
E) Requesting that all caregivers call the patient by their preferred pronoun

ANSWER KEY

1. D	14. A	27. C	40. A, D, E
2. B	15. B	28. C	41. A
3. A	16. C	29. C	42. A, B, D, F
4. A	17. A, D, E	30. D	43. B
5. D	18. C	31. A, C, D, E	44. A
6. B	19. D	32. B	45. C
7. B	20. B	33. A	46. B
8. C	21. C	34. A, B, C	47. D
9. A	22. B	35. B, C	48. A, B, D
10. A	23. A, B, E	36. D	49. A, B, D, E
11. C	24. C	37. A	50. A, B, E
12. C	25. B	38. B	
13. D	26. D	39. D	

NCLEX Next Generation Questions

1. Exhibit item

Mr. Blake is an 80-year-old patient who presents status post-fall. He is awake with a contusion noted on the right elbow with no active bleeding. His past medical history is significant for hypertension.

He lives with his wife and dog. He completed high school and worked as a contractor before retiring at 65.

Vital signs: BP 118/70; HR 78; O2 saturation 96%; RR 18; SLUMS 14

When reviewing Mr. Blake's intake note, which item does the nurse recognize requires follow-up?

A) SLUMS 14

B) HR 78

C) Contusion right elbow

D) O2 saturation 96%

Answer/Rationale: A

A SLUMS score of 14 in those who completed high school likely indicates dementia. Further evaluation will be required to determine the patient's mental status, as it may increase his risk for future falls. An HR of 78 and O2 saturation of 96% are within normal limits. A nonbleeding contusion of the elbow may require further observation but is not the priority.

2. Exhibit

Hailey, who is 8 years old, presents for her annual physical. Today, she weighs 70 pounds and measures 53 inches. Use the growth chart to determine her weight-percentile.

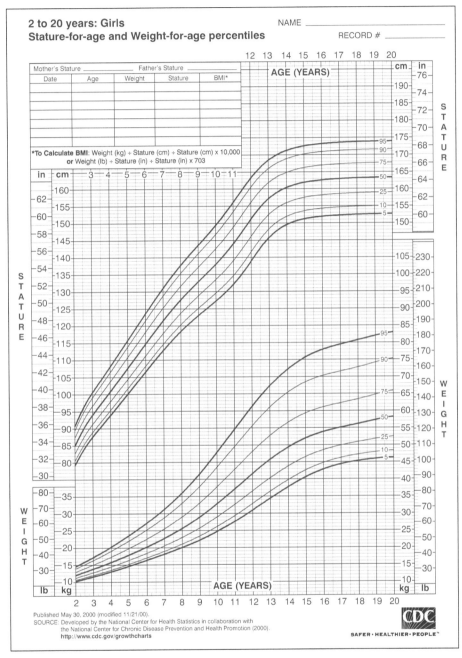

A) 90th percentile

B) 75th percentile

C) 50th percentile

D) 30th percentile

Answer/Rationale: A

The patient's gender, age, and weight place her in the 90th percentile.

3. Hot spot

A patient who has recently experienced a stroke is having difficulty with coordination. Select the area of the brain that has most likely been affected. *Place an 'x' on the image in the correct location.*

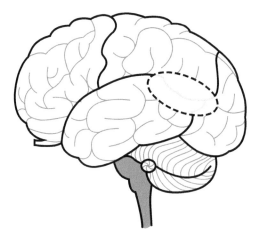

Answer/Rationale:

The cerebellum, located at the base of the brain, is responsible for coordination.

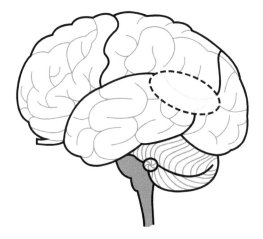

4. Hot spot

When assessing a patient with suspect left ventricular enlargement, the nurse palpates for the position of the point of maximal impulse (PMI). Where does the nurse place their fingers to palpate the PMI? *Place an 'x' on the image in the correct location.*

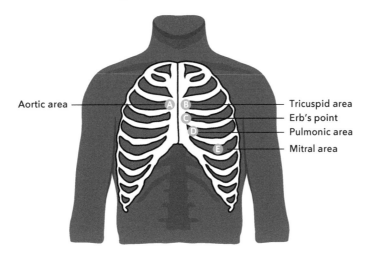

Answer/Rationale:

The PMI can be felt in the same location as mitral auscultation, the 5th/6th intercostal space at the left midclavicular line.

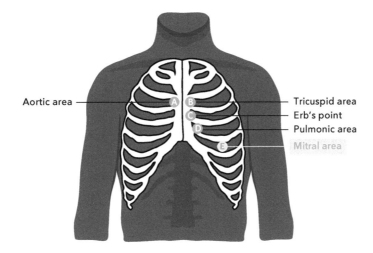

5. Matrix

A 65-year-old patient with a history of chronic bronchitis for 15 years presents to the emergency department for evaluation. When performing the physical assessment, which findings does the nurse expect to find? *Place an 'x' in the correlating box to indicate if the finding is expected or unexpected.*

Assessment Finding	Expected	Not Expected
1:1 A-P transverse diameter		
Oxygenation saturation 93%		
Respiratory rate 28		
Rhonchi upon auscultation		

Answer/Rationale:

Assessment Finding	Expected	Not Expected
1:1 A-P transverse diameter	X	
Oxygenation saturation 93%	X	
Respiratory rate 28		X
Rhonchi upon auscultation		X

An A-P transverse ratio of 1:1 indicate barrel chest. While this is not a normal finding, it is anticipated in patients with longstanding chronic bronchitis as pulmonary remodeling takes place. In a patient with no disease, a 1:2 ratio is expected. An oxygen saturation of 93% is an expected finding in chronic bronchitis, as patients live in a hypoxic, hypercapnic state. In patients with no history of respiratory disease, an O2 saturation of > 95% should be expected. A respiratory rate of 28 is elevated and may indicate an exacerbation of chronic bronchitis. Rhonchi indicate increased mucous in the airways and might also be a sign of exacerbation.

6. Hot spot

A 22-year-old patient presents to the urgent care clinic with complaints of fever and abdominal pain. She is concerned she might have appendicitis. Pain felt in which area of the abdomen most strongly suggests inflammation of the appendix? *Place an 'x' in the correct region.*

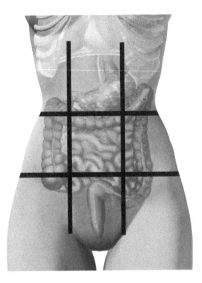

Answer/Rationale:

The appendix is located in the right iliac region of the abdomen. Pain related to inflammation of the appendix is most often felt in this area.

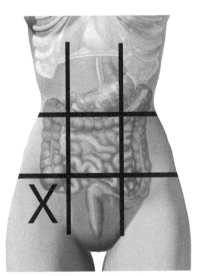

7. Cloze

A patient whose LMP was on July 17th, 2023, presents for complaints of abdominal fullness. During her exam, the cervix is noted to have a bluish color consistent with ___1___. Additionally, the cervix has softened, indicating a positive ___2___. A positive urine ___3___ determines the patient is pregnant. The nurse calculates the estimated date of delivery to be ___4___.

Complete the sentence using the following options.

1. Chadwick's sign, Goodell's sign, Hegar's sign
2. Chadwick's sign, Goodell's sign, Hegar's sign
3. HCG, protein, ketone
4. April 24th, 2024; March 3rd, 2024; February 3rd, 2024

Answer/Rationale:

1. **Chadwick's sign:** The bluish discoloration of the cervix that develops after six to eight weeks of pregnancy.
2. **Goodell's sign:** The softening of the cervix as a consequence of increased hormone production.
3. **HCG:** Human chorionic gonadotropin is a hormone detectable in blood and urine that rises with pregnancy.
4. **April 24th, 2024:** Nagel's rule is used to calculate the estimated date of delivery.

   July – 3 months = April

   17 + 7 days = 24

   Next year 2024

8. Extended multiple response

The nurse is evaluating a new skin lesion. Which qualities of the lesion increase the nurse's suspicion of malignancy? *(Select all that apply)*

A) Irregular borders
B) Diameter 9 mm
C) Brown coloration
D) Ragged borders
E) Lesion symmetry
F) Stable appearance since last visit

Answer: A, B, D

9. Matrix

A patient is diagnosed with a thyroid goiter. They are undergoing further evaluation for possible thyroid dysfunction. Which signs and symptoms should the nurse associate with hypothyroidism or hyperthyroidism? *Place an 'x' in the matrix to indicate if the sign/symptom is found in hypothyroidism or hyperthyroidism.*

Sign/Symptom	Hypothyroidism	Hyperthyroidism
Weight gain		
Cold intolerance		
Heart palpitations		
Dry skin		
Tremor		

Answer:

Sign/Symptom	Hypothyroidism	Hyperthyroidism
Weight gain	X	
Cold intolerance	X	
Heart palpitations		X
Dry skin	X	
Tremor		X

10. Extended multiple response

The nurse caring for a transgender patient notes bruising on the patient's wrists and back. Which assessment does the nurse prioritize for this patient?

   A) Screen for IPV
   B) Assess the blood pressure
   C) Administer a PHQ-9 questionnaire
   D) Inspect for equal chest expansion
   E) Palpate the point of maximal impulse (PMI)

Answer: A